Table of Contents

Introduction

Modern lifestyle has a great influence on the risk of overweight in humans. The epidemic of overweight is a consequence of the modern way of life. Unlike our ancestors, who were engaged mainly in physical labor and ate natural homemade food, we live in a period of technological progress and fast food. Due to technological progress, the share of physical labor in the last 100 years decreased from 95% to 5%.

Nowadays, there are overweight people among us who suffer from various disorders of the digestive tract, high blood pressure, diabetes and many other diseases, the occurrence of which is associated with uncontrolled food intake.

What is good and what is bad? I need hardly say that our nutrition is necessary to maintain our lives. In addition, healthy eating is one of the fundamental moments of our healthy lifestyle and, consequently, the preservation and strengthening of our health. This significant and constantly acting factor ensures adequate growth and development of our body. Rational healthy nutrition provides us with adequate physical and neuropsychological development, increases resistance to infectious diseases and resistance to unfavorable environmental conditions.

Recently, people are trying to pay more attention to their health. We choose food more carefully because our body must receive the necessary compounds like proteins, fats, carbohydrates, vitamins and mineral nutrients. Now we already know that the diet should be balanced and serve as the source of all these components. If you are worried about your weight, health, and nutrition, you should know that you are ready to change your usual life and give up the harmful food. Let us get rid of the overweight together.

Today, I offer to you a keto cookbook, which is your chance to lose weight fast! The ketogenic diet is one of the famous ways to achieve effective results in losing weight and reduce the risk factors of various diseases. Nevertheless, before starting a diet you should check the condition of all organs and body systems. Otherwise, the harm of a diet can be irreparable.

Good luck!

What is The Ketogenic Diet

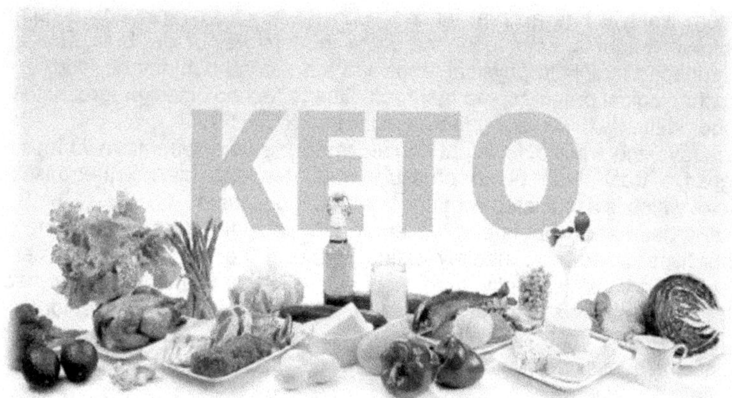

There are many scientific data indicating that ketogenic diet is not only a highly effective way to reduce weight but also shows more stable results compared to traditional low-fat systems requiring severe calorie restriction. It has been shown that people using a ketogenic diet lose 2.2 times more pounds of excess weight than volunteers who used a low-fat diet with severe calorie restriction.

If the truth be known the keto diet which limits carbohydrates and allows fats have been clinically tested in the 1920s. The medical faculty who treated patients, who suffered CNS system diseases, often prescribed courses of the keto diet, which significantly limited the production of insulin and other hormones that affect the activity of the central nervous system and brain. In addition, doctors for various diseases, for instance, diabetes, cancer, epilepsy and Alzheimer's disease, prescribed this keto diet. Now let us understand how the ketogenic diet works and what biological processes underlie it.

Glucose is the main food for our cells. It is stored in the liver and muscles in the form of a complex carbohydrate glycogen, which provides a stable level of glucose in the blood and gives energy for muscle activity. Glycogen stores are limited, so our cells start using other sources of energy, such as proteins and fats, in conditions of starvation or insufficient supply of carbohydrates with food. During gluconeogenesis, new glucose molecules are synthesized also from their structural components.

When the glucose is reducing the in the blood, the cells of organs and tissues are experiencing energy shortage. The oxidation of fatty acids is a laborious process, and the nervous tissue is generally unable to oxidize fatty acids, so our liver facilitates the use of these acids by tissues, in advance oxidizing them to acetic acid and converting them into ketonic bodies. The incentive for the formation of ketone bodies is the flow of a large number of fatty acids into our liver.

In addition, the oxidation process of fatty acids is formed such ketone bodies acetoacetic acid, beta-hydroxybutyric acid, and acetone. They serve as an alternative source of energy for our cells when glucose for some reason is not available. If the body is fed mainly from fats, the concentration of ketone bodies in the blood increases significantly. They cross the hematoencephalic barrier and give energy to the brain, providing about two-thirds of its needs. Under normal conditions, the brain is powered by glucose, that is, ketosis is a mechanism of adaptation that allows a person to survive. Ketones are used by muscle and other tissues and even appear in the urine.

HOW DOES KETOSIS WORK?

TRADITIONAL DIET: HIGHER CARB

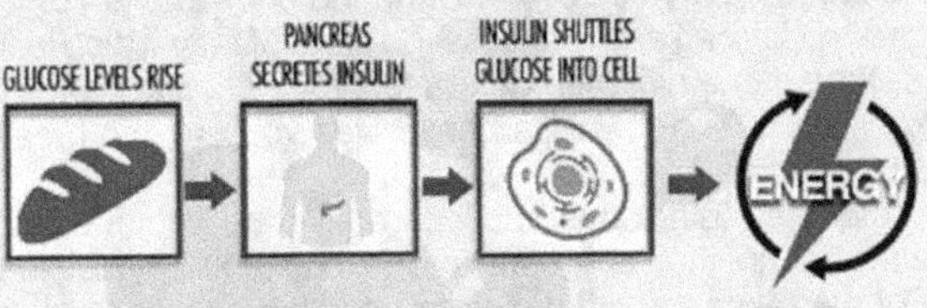

KETO DIET: HIGHER FAT

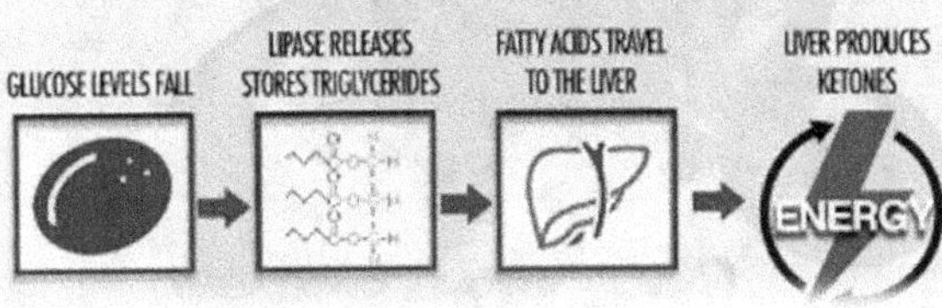

In such a manner ketosis is a metabolic state that occurs when the amount of carbohydrate in your diet is so low that the body is forced to use as energy fatty acids and metabolism of ketone bodies. That sounds simple, but let us look at this process to understand why our body enters a state of ketosis.

To function our body needs a sufficient amount of energy in the form of ATP. ATP is a universal source of energy for all biochemical processes occurring in living systems. A person needs about 1800 kcal per day to produce enough ATP to maintain viability. At the same time, our brain requires about 400 kcal per day and uses glucose as energy. This means that a person needs to consume 100 g of glucose per day only to maintain the normal functioning of the brain. What does that have to do with ketosis? When we use the keto diet, we eliminate almost all carbohydrates from our diet. That means we deprive our brains of glucose. Nevertheless, we need glucose for brain function. Fortunately, the liver stores glucose in the form of glycogen and can give a small amount of it to our brain to work. Our liver can store an average of 100-120 grams of glucose. In the condition of a critical shortage of carbohydrates for the brain, liver gives us the opportunity to work normally during the day. However, the supply of glucose in the liver does not resume quickly. In addition, carbohydrates are needed not only the brain, so we have health problems.

Our muscles are also a huge repository of glucose. They contain 400 to 500 grams of glucose as glycogen form. However, glycogen stores are not intended to feed our brain. Unfortunately, our muscles cannot break down glycogen and put it into the flow of blood to supply our brains eventually. Our muscles do not have an enzyme that can break down glycogen (glucose-6-phosphate dehydrogenase). In the absence of carbohydrates, the liver begins to produce ketone bodies that are transferred by a flow of blood to our brain and other tissues that do not use fat as energy. Gradually, with a regular shortage of carbohydrates, the body reaches the state of ketosis. This process takes place constantly and the level of ketone bodies

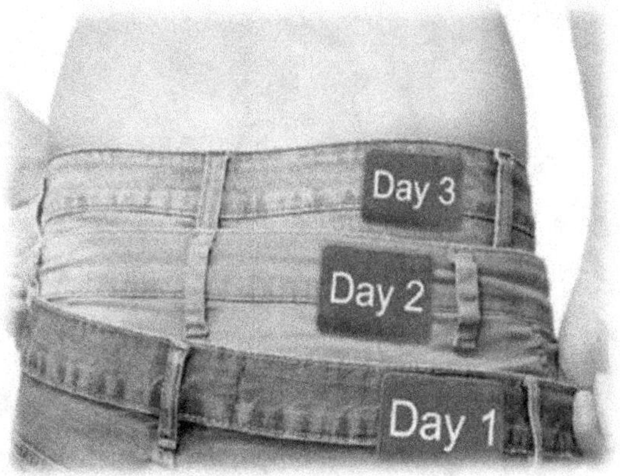

increases markedly in the blood. In the state of ketosis, ketone bodies are produced in large quantities, and they are used as fuel by our body. Ketones serve as an alternative energy source for the body, which uses at a lowered level of glucose in the blood.

As mentioned before, using such diet, the human body uses fat as fuel. Under such conditions, the level of insulin in the blood becomes very low, and the consumption of fats increases dramatically. Now the human body can easily access the store of fats, which leads to the intensive use of them. Under the ketone diet, you do not feel food cravings and you have a continuous supply of energy source. The fewer carbohydrates you eat, the greater the impact on weight and blood sugar levels.

The ketogenic diet is a very strict diet. It includes a low carbohydrate content and is therefore very effective. The healthy menu that collected in this cookbook significantly increases the physical endurance of the human body, providing constant access to all the energy that produces from the stores of fats. In order to make the ketogenic diet really simple and pleasant, you need to learn new useful recipes that described in this book. Here you will find fifty recipes that could help you choose dishes that contain low levels of carbohydrates.

How can it benefit you?

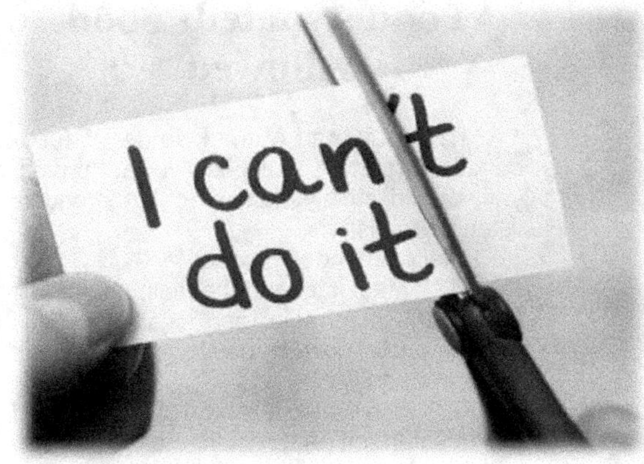

Health is the most precious treasure that, along with life, is given to us free. Maybe that is why so often we do not appreciate its importance and significance. For most of us, investing in health seems too long and tedious a process. Moreover, it never gives us full confidence that the time and effort spent will ever come back to us as a reward. The overweight problems frequently leads to serious health consequences such as cardiovascular diseases, mainly heart disease and stroke, and diabetes, muscular-skeletal injuries, such as osteoarthritis, and some cancers, for instance cancer of the endometrium, breast death and colorectal carcinoma. These conditions cause premature death or disability. For these reasons, people who has overweight decide to change their lives, improve health, and increase the possibility of fulfilling themselves in community. However, this task is not for everyone.

You should believe me that weight loss will be unreal if you do not have a good incentive. To understand this, ask yourself one question, namely what benefits can be derived from weight loss? If you cannot answer this question, then you do not have a good incentive for weight loss. Therefore, you should not struggle with excess weight. Such an attempt to lose weight, not having a clear goal will not benefit you, and will be a waste of time. Nevertheless, if you still have a desire, then you will not be difficult to lose weight. The most important thing is to set yourself a goal! What goal? I will tell you!

1. Improve your health and well-being (reduce shortness of breath, reduce high blood pressure, joint pain, spine pain, improve carbohydrate and lipid metabolism).
2. The expansion of everyday physical capabilities (easier to walk, climb stairs, work in the garden to play and run with children).
3. Reducing the psychological problems associated with being overweight. Increase your self-esteem.
4. Improving the appearance (attractive appearance, the ability to dress nice and fashionable, go to the gym, sauna, swimming pool, and beach).
5. Improvement of family and sexual relations.
6. Increase fertility and reduce the risk of transmission to children of harmful lifestyles that lead to obesity and other diseases.
7. Improvement of professional opportunities, including professional growth.
8. You will be able to buy clothes cheaper! It is no secret that large size clothing is more expensive.
9. You will learn about human physiology and weight loss process. Agree, if you know that for burning one bar of chocolate you need to run for 4 hours you will be more careful with the choice of food.
10. You will like yourself. You will see a reflection in the mirror that pleases you.
11. You should remember that your body is entirely up to you. Do not be lazy!

Agree, for the sake of these pleasant moments should work hard for months or even years! You must try keto. Who knows perhaps and your way of life will radically change to the best for you!

KETO Food Pyramid

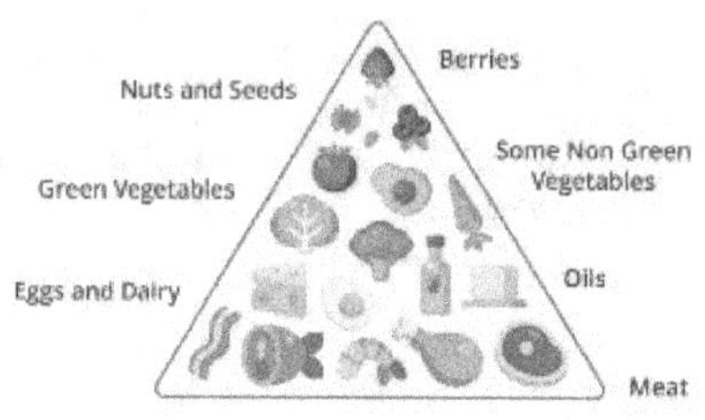

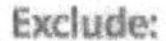

Exclude:

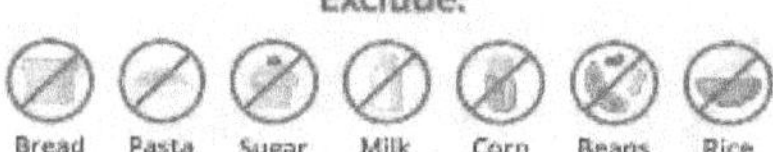

Food Avoided/ Food Allowed

The main part of the keto diet is food-containing protein. For effective fat burning, you should strictly adhere to the products listed in this list.

Recommended product:

1. Meat is one of the main sources of food rich in protein and vitamins. It is recommended to use poultry, beef, rabbits and even pork;

2. Fish is also a source of proteins and polyunsaturated fatty acids. Eating redfish, cod, herring, flounder, capelin, halibut and tuna will balance the diet;

3. Seafood (mussels, squid, crab, shrimps, and oysters) is rich not only in protein but also in nutrients. Also, these substances are well absorbed by the body;

4. Eggs are a product rich in vitamins and minerals. Chicken and quail eggs are important components of the keto diet;

5. Nuts are suitable as a small snack between the main meals (almonds, walnuts, hazelnuts, and pistachios)

6. Non-fat dairy products are rich in calcium, vitamins, and minerals (cottage cheese, cheese, yogurt, skim milk and kefir);

7. Vegetables are a useful and low-calorie product rich in fiber. However, their intake should be limited. Because some of them contain a large number of carbohydrates. You should use for your diet green salad, spinach, radish, cucumbers, zucchini, and cabbage.

8. Fruits allow the use of unsweetened apples, grapefruit, and oranges.

The following list contains the strictly prohibited to use products:

Prohibited products:

1. Cereals (rice, buckwheat, oatmeal, millet, pearl);
2. Confectionery (cakes, chocolate, marshmallow, waffles);
3. Bakery products (bread, loaf);
4. Sugar;
5. Vegetables with a high content of carbohydrates (potatoes, Yam, corn, parsley, onion, garlic);
6. Carbonated drinks;
7. Sweet fruits (bananas, grapes, mango, persimmon).

The optimal amount of carbohydrates per day should not exceed 50 grams. You should also drink plenty of fluids, namely 1.5-2 liters of water a day. The approximate ratio of proteins, fats, and carbohydrates will look like this: 25 % — 70% — 5%.

Healthy nutrition is one of the basic conditions of human existence, and the problem of nutrition is one of the main problems of human culture. Doubtless, healthy nutrition is the most significant part of our health. For this reason, I recommend you the keto diet as a famous and effective way to quickly lose weight and reduce the risk factors of various diseases. This is why my main task was to collect as many recipes as possible for the ketogenic menu. Another good thing about keto diet is that it has a positive effect on the hardiness of a person and life activity, and determines the duration and usefulness of life quality. I wish you with pleasure to pass the way to ideal health, optimal weight, and inexhaustible vital energy.

What is a Crock-Pot?

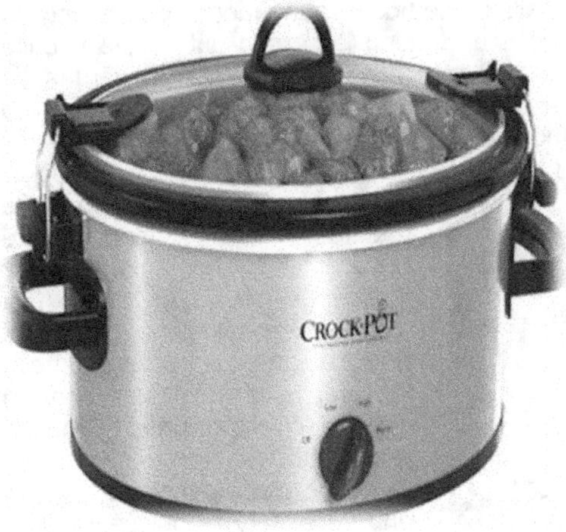

Speed is a symbol of modern life. We are in a hurry, overtaking each other. We only make a stop in the kitchen. Here the rush is not necessary because each dish requires attention and reverent attitude. Based on these requirements, develop such equipment, which exempts modern cooks from the need to participate in the long process of cooking. One of these improvements is a kitchen technique called a crock pot. The purpose of the crock pot is to prepare dishes, recipes of which are designed for slow cooking. With its help, you can cook and stew a variety of dishes, such as stuffed cabbage, large pieces of meat, pilaf, cabbage, and a variety of porridge. Those who are fond of canning, as it is very convenient to cook jam on a low heat, will appreciate the crock pot.

To cook a dish with the help of the crock pot, it is enough to put all the necessary ingredients in the pot and set the desired program. Cooking takes place at a temperature not exceeding 80 degrees, so the food does not burn, does not require constant stirring and will not boil. When the food is ready, the appliance will automatically enter the heating mode.

This simple principle of the crock pot is ensured by its technical characteristics. The crock pot is a device consisting of a container with heating elements, which is inserted into the pot for cooking. The volume of the pot varies between different models from three to six liters. Usually, the slow cooker is designed for three programs, the name of which depends on the model and manufacturer. The maximum cooking time of individual models of up to 12 hours.

It is noteworthy that the removable crock pot and can be used in the microwave oven, as it is ceramic. The design of the crock pot has a 3D-heating function, in which the products in the pan are heated not only from the bottom but also from the sides. Technical characteristics of the crockpot can surprise anyone. The capacity of the kitchen appliances is 350 watts. The transparent lid is made of impact-resistant glass. The body of the crock

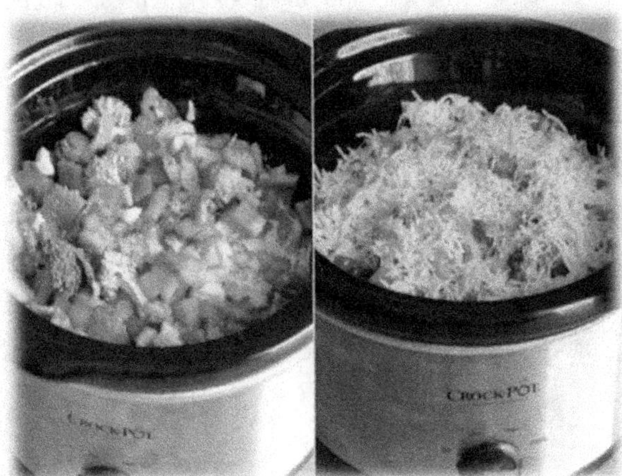

pot is made of stainless steel, and the bottom is equipped with a rubberized stand that protects the surface of the table from heating. The handle of the crock pot also will not heat.

Almost all models of crock pots have electronic control. The body has a built-in display, which is very convenient to control the cooking process by selecting the desired program.

Depending on the placement of heating elements, there are two types of the crock pots. In the crock pots of the first type, the heating elements are built into the walls of the body, so the food warms evenly. In the crock pots of the second type the process of heating is carried out by the heating elements located on the bottom of the tank, so the cooking process is even slower than in the first case. When working with such models, you need to remember that every time you open the lid, you need to increase the cooking time for 20 minutes.

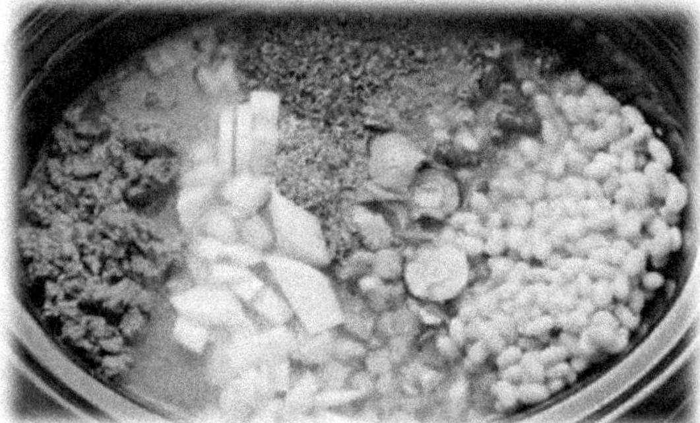

The choice of crock pots should be done taking into account the above features and your taste preferences. The most popular today are crock pots of the first type. When choosing the crock pots, pay attention to the volume of the pot and maximum cooking time, which is designed especially for this model.

The crock pot is a wonderful and necessary technique for your kitchen. It helps to realize the dream of each of us about healthy and useful food, and the cooking process will not take much of your time and will not be tedious.

Stewing dishes in the crock pot is perhaps the gentlest way of cooking products. The temperature during cooking by this method rarely rises above 80-90°C, which allows maximum preservation of vitamins and minerals. It is not just stewing food, but slow cooking for a long time, which can reach 10-12 hours! The advantages of this method of cooking are obvious.

There are no special difficulties in dealing with the crock pot, but a few rules still need to be remembered. For example, do not put frozen foods in the pot, it is better to defrost them in advance. You should cut vegetables into pieces of the same size. Before laying the meat in the pot, be sure to cut off all visible fat from it because it does not evaporate and does not melt with such gentle heat treatment. Meat can be pre-fried to preserve flavor and at the same time to drown excess fat. Onions can also fry before putting in the crock pot, but if there is no time, you can cook vegetables without frying. When cooking, accurately calculate the amount of water, as the liquid does not evaporate.

For best results, fill the crock pot at least halfway, but leave at least 5 cm before the lid. All products should be almost covered with liquid (broth, sauce, gravy, etc.). While modifying the usual recipes for the crock pot, remember that the cooking time should be increased by four times. Remember that vegetables are cooked the longest, and then put the poultry and meat, and the seafood is prepared the fastest. Therefore, vegetables should be at the bottom of the pot. During cooking, try not to open the lid, as the temperature drops, and cooking time increases by 10-20 minutes with each opening of the lid.

Additionally, when installing a crock pot in your kitchen, remember that steam comes out of it, so you need to think about safety. Make sure that there is free space around the pot so that steam can evaporate while cooking. You should definitely read the instructions for the use of crock pot. Please note that different types of crock pot have different functions and instructions for cleaning and maintaining the appliance. Follow the safety technique!

Healthy vegetable dishes

1.Stew with vegetables

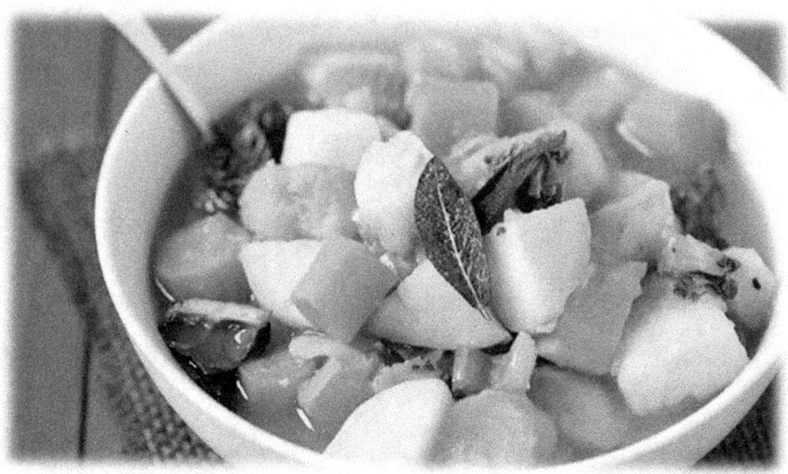

Ingredients (10 servings):

- 200 g of broccoli
- 200 g of zucchini
- 4 cups of clear vegetable soup
- 3 cloves of garlic
- 1.5 teaspoon of curry powder
- 1,5 teaspoon of ground cumin
- 1,5 teaspoon of ground ginger
- 3 tablespoons of fresh coriander
- 1/3 cup of cashew

Cooking instruction:

As a first step, you should place the sliced zucchini, broccoli, and garlic in a crock pot. Then add curry, cumin, ginger and pour all the ingredients into the clear vegetable soup. Stir well. After that, you should close the crock pot and cook the stew on low power for 4.5-5 hours or on strong power for 2-2.5 hours. Well done! Then add the chopped fresh herbs. Now you should mix all ingredients thoroughly and serve the stew with vegetables with cashew.

Enjoy your meal!

2.Mexican vegetable stew

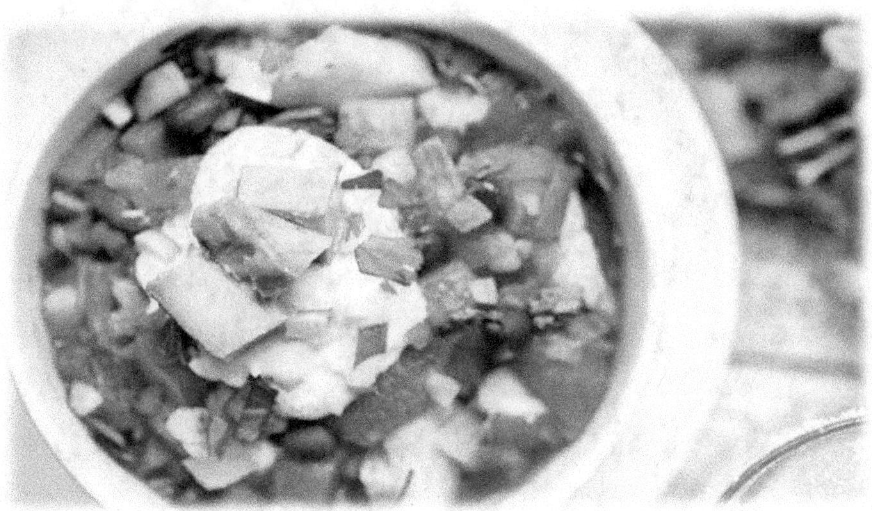

Ingredients (7 servings):

- 150 g of sliced tomatoes
- lime juice to taste
- 150 g of sliced pepper
- 150 g of any fresh herbs
- 150 g of asparagus
- 2 cloves of garlic
- 4 cups of clear vegetable soup

Cooking instruction:

In the first instance, you should place the sliced pepper, asparagus, sliced tomatoes and garlic in a crock pot. Then add salt and pour all the ingredients into the clear vegetable soup. Stir well. After that, you should close the crock pot and cook the vegetable on low power for 4.5-5 hours or on strong power for 2-2.5 hours. Well done! Now you can add lime juice to taste. Stir all ingredients well. After that, you should add the chopped fresh herbs. Stir thoroughly again. Serve Mexican vegetable stew immediately.

Enjoy your meal!

3.Vegetable stew with tuna

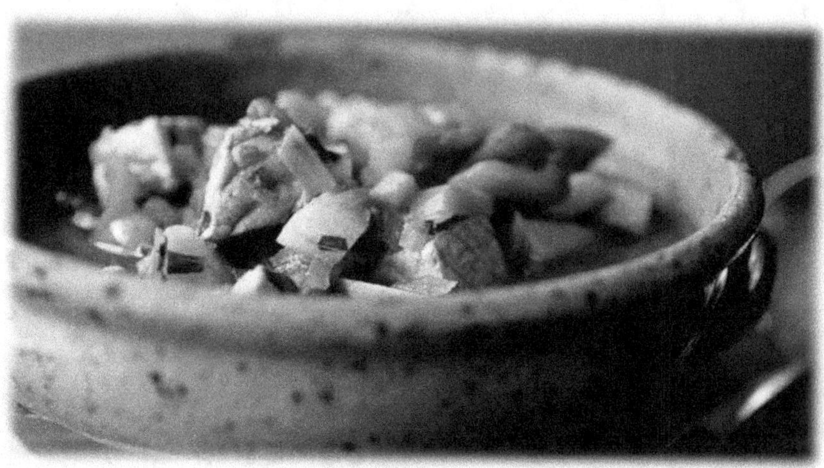

Ingredients (13 servings):

- 30 g of olive oil
- 1 onion
- 1 clove of garlic
- 200 g of finely chopped tomatoes
- 150 g of vegetable or fish broth
- 1 teaspoon of paprika
- 1/2 teaspoon of chili pepper
- sweet pepper to taste
- sprig of fresh rosemary
- 10 g of Bay leaf
- 450 g of tuna fillet
- salt to taste
- black pepper to taste

Cooking instruction:

As a first step, you should heat the olive oil in a large pan. Then add the onion and fry for 10 minutes. The onions should be soft. After that add garlic, broth, tomatoes, and sprinkle with paprika and chili. Stir well and bring the mass to boil, and then pass this mass to the bowl of the crock pot. Then add tuna fillet, sweet pepper, rosemary, and Bay leaf and mix well all ingredients. Now you should close the crock pot and cook vegetables for about 2-2.5 hours. Now you can add salt and pepper to taste. You can now add the tuna pieces. Well done! Cover the crock pot with a lid and cook the dish for another 15-20 minutes, until the fish is cooked. Serve immediately.
Enjoy your meal!

4.Stew with pumpkin and Turkey

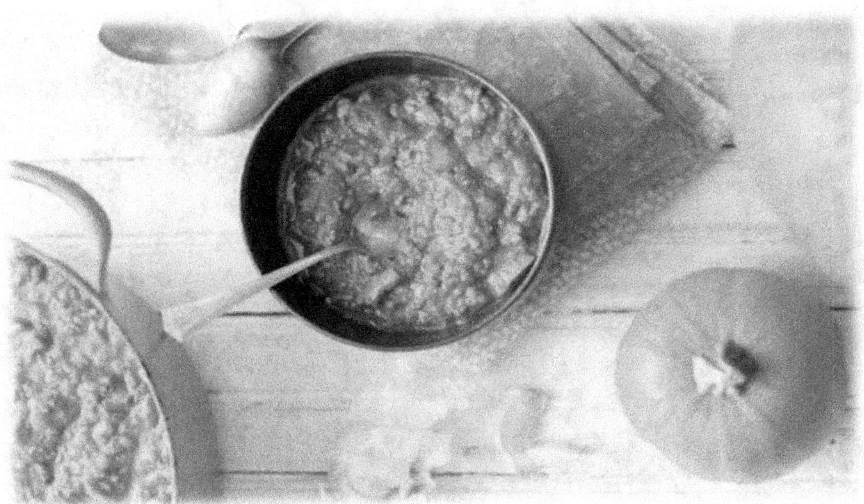

Ingredients (6 servings):

- 700 g of turkey
- 900 g of pumpkin
- 1 onion
- 400 g of tomatoes
- 3-4 sprigs of parsley
- vegetable oil

Cooking instruction:

In the first instance, you should remove the skin from the turkey. Then you should peel the pumpkin, remove all seeds, and cut into cubes 2.5 cm. Now slice the onion into half rings and chop the parsley. Now you can oil the bowl of crock pot with oil. Then place all the prepared ingredients, except parsley. You should cook the dish on low power for 4.5-5 hours or on strong power for 2-2.5 hours. Well done! Now you should get the meat out of the pot. After that, you need to remove the meat from the bones and cut it into small pieces. Now place the meat on the ingredients and mix well. Before serving, decorate the dish with chopped parsley. Serve immediately.
Enjoy your meal!

5.Bell peppers with meat

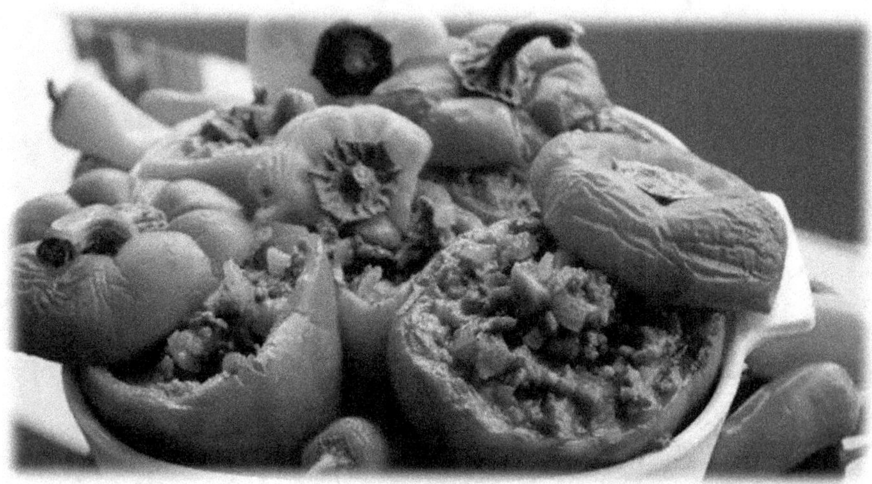

Ingredients (9 servings):

- 8 sweet peppers
- 700 g of mince of beef
- 250 g of tomato sauce
- 1 onion
- 2 cloves garlic
- any grated cheese
- salt to taste
- 1 cup of water or clear vegetable soup
- pepper to taste

Cooking instruction:

As a first step, you should make sweet pepper cups. After that, you should remove all seeds from the pepper. Now, you can peel the onion and garlic and finely chop them. Mix the minced meat, pepper, onion, garlic, and tomato sauce. By the way, instead of beef meat, you can use any minced meat. Then you should add salt, pepper to taste and stir the minced meat well. Next, you can fill the peppers with minced meat and sprinkle with grated cheese. After that, you should place the peppers in the crock pot and add water or clear vegetable soup. After that, cover the crock pot with a lid tightly and cook the peppers for 6-7 hours. Well done! Serve immediately.

Enjoy your meal!

6.Stew with chicken and vegetables

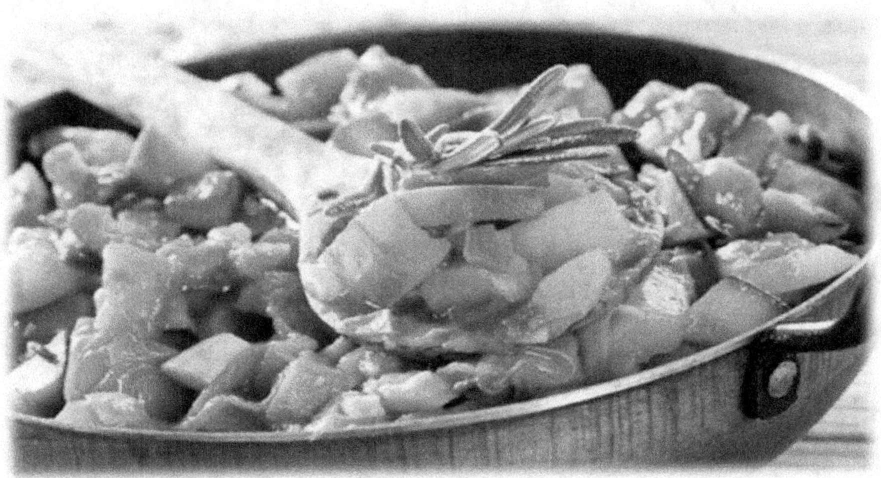

Ingredients (12 servings):

- 500 g of chicken fillet
- 2 sweet peppers
- 1 tomato
- fresh herbs to taste
- 200 g of sliced zucchini
- 1 onion
- 2 cloves garlic
- 1 tablespoon of chili powder
- 2 teaspoons of cumin
- 1 teaspoon of paprika
- 2 cups of water or clear vegetable soup

Cooking instruction:

In the first instance, you should remove all seeds from pepper and cut them into slices. Then peel and chop onion and garlic. After that cut tomato and zucchini. In addition, you should add 1 tablespoon of chili powder, 2 teaspoons of cumin and 1 teaspoon of paprika. Stir all sliced vegetables thoroughly. Now, you can place all ingredients in the crock pot. If you want, you can cut the chicken fillet into a straw. Next, you should put the chicken fillet and 2 cups of water or clear vegetable soup in the crock pot. After that, you can cover the crock pot with a lid and cook for 7-8 hours. Well done! Do not forget to decorate the dish with fresh herbs to taste. Serve immediately!
    Enjoy your meal!

7.Vegetable sauce

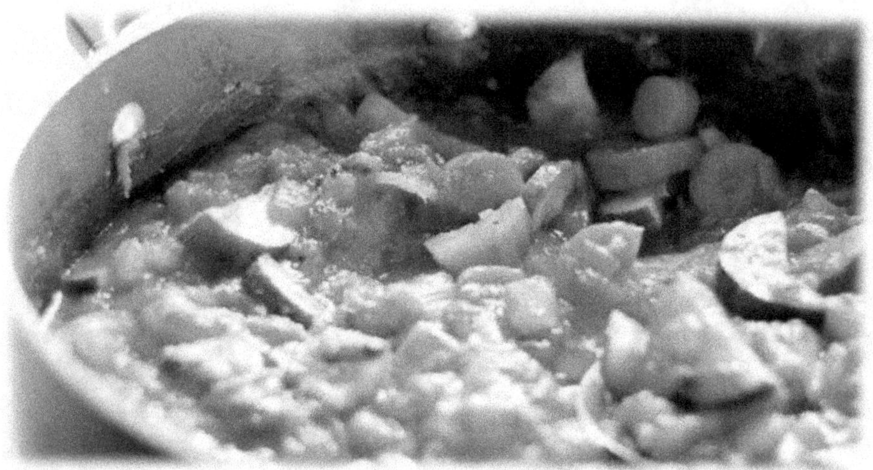

Ingredients (11 servings):

- 2 onions
- 1 celery root
- 1 sweet pepper
- 4 cloves of garlic
- 150 g of vegetable marrow
- 4 tablespoons of tomato paste
- a bunch of parsley
- a bunch of dills
- 1 cup of water or clear vegetable soup
- salt to taste
- black pepper to taste

Cooking instruction:

As a first step, you should finely chop the celery root, sweet pepper, onions, vegetable marrow and cloves of garlic. After that place all chopped vegetables in the crock pot and add four tablespoons of tomato paste. Now, you should stir all ingredients well. Then pour a cup of water or clear vegetable soup and add a bunch of parsley and bunch of dills. Mix the vegetable sauce thoroughly. After that, add salt and black pepper to taste and stir well again. Next, you should cover the crock pot with a lid and cook the vegetable sauce on low power for 4.5-5 hours or on strong power for 2-2.5 hours. Well done! Then add the chopped fresh herbs to your taste. Serve the dish immediately!

Enjoy your meal!

8.Vegetarian vegetable spread

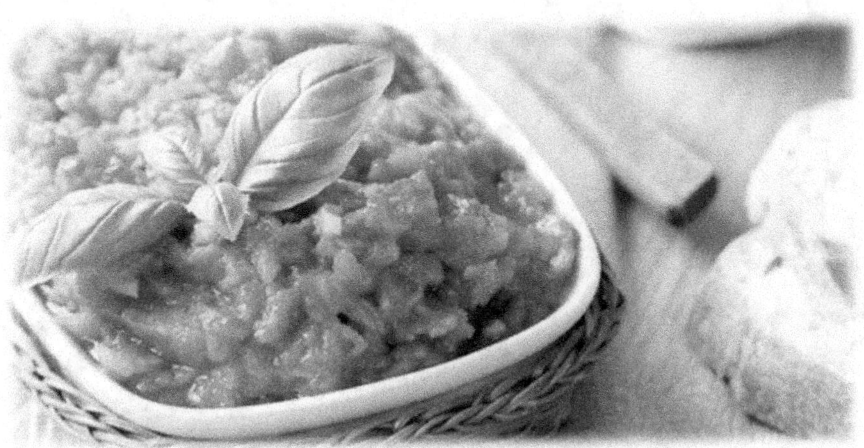

Ingredients (11 servings):

- 500 g of eggplant
- 500 kg of tomato
- 1 kg of sweet pepper
- 300 g of onion
- 100 g of vegetable oil
- 1 bunch of parsley
- 1 bunch of dill
- black pepper to taste
- 100 g of garlic or to taste
- salt to taste

Cooking instruction:

In the first instance, you should place the chopped onions, and the sliced tomatoes in the blender and grind them thoroughly. Then pour the tomato mass into the crock pot and cook on low power for 4.5-5 hours or on strong power for 2-2.5 hours. After that, place sweet pepper in boiling water for three minutes, and then put them out and peel. Now, you can grind the sweet pepper in the blender. Next, you should cut eggplants and simmer them until a ruddy color appears. Once again, blend all the ingredients in the blender. Then mix the onions, eggplants, dill, tomatoes, parsley, and pepper in a crock pot. In addition, add the pepper and salt to taste. After that, you should cook the vegetable sauce on low power for 2.5 - 3 hours or on strong power for 1-1.5 hours. Well done!
Enjoy your meal!

9.Vegetables stewed with spices

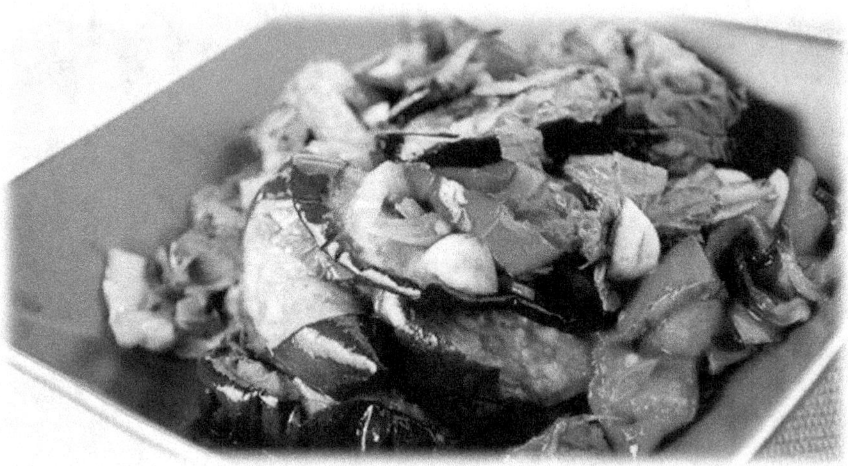

Ingredients (13 servings):

- ¼ of eggplant
- ¼ of cabbage
- 1 tomato
- garlic to taste
- fresh herbs to taste
- 50 g of butter
- 100 g of sour cream
- 100 g of grated cheese
- 150 ml of water or clear vegetable soup
- 1/6 teaspoon of ground black pepper
- 1/4 teaspoon of ground coriander
- 1/4 teaspoon of ground ginger
- 10 g of bay leaf

Cooking instruction:

As a first step, you should place layers of sliced tomato, cabbage and the eggplant and garlic on the bottom of the crock pot. After that, add 150 ml of water or clear vegetable soup and a bay leaf. You should not stir ingredients. Cover the pot with a lid and cook the vegetables on low power for 4.5-5 hours or on strong power for 2-2.5 hours. Well done! Then add butter, spices, cheese, and sour cream. Stir the ingredients thoroughly. After that, you should place all ingredients in the frying pan and cook them for 3 minutes. Serve immediately!

Enjoy your meal!

Fish and seafood

10.Italian soup with salmon

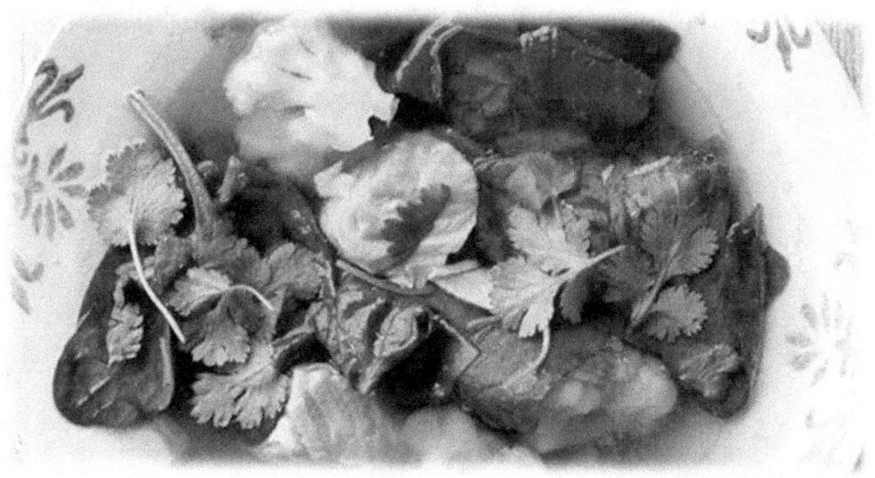

Ingredients (8 servings):

- 400 g of salmon
- 100 g of spinach
- 100 g of cauliflower
- 1 onion
- parsley to taste
- black pepper to taste
- vegetable oil
- salt to taste

Cooking instruction:

In the first instance, you should put the fish in the crock pot. Then add cold water, and cook the fish for about 2-2.5 hours. After that, remove the bones from the boiled fish, and then divide the meat into medium-sized pieces. After chopping the onion, red pepper into small cubes. The sliced vegetables fry in vegetable oil. Then place the vegetables in the broth and bring the soup to a boil. Boil all the ingredients for 10 to 12 minutes. Then add the chopped spinach to the pan with the fish pieces. Add salt and pepper to taste. Stir the broth thoroughly and add the paprika. Bring the broth to a boil. Well done!

Enjoy your meal!

11.Stews with seafood

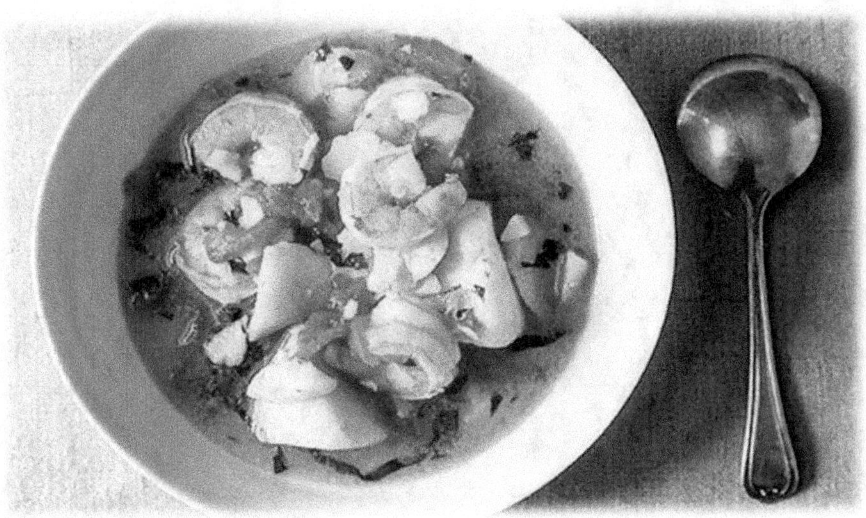

Ingredients (10 servings):

- 450 g of mussels (shelled)
- 240 g of scallops
- 240 g of medium size shrimps (shelled)
- 400 g of tomatoes
- 1.5 tablespoons of olive oil
- 0.5 cups of sliced onion
- 1.5 teaspoon of chopped garlic
- 0.25 teaspoons of dried red pepper
- 0.5 cups of fish broth
- 0.25 cups of chopped fresh parsley

Cooking instruction:

In the first instance, you should heat the olive oil in a deep frying pan. Then put the onion, garlic and crushed red pepper. You should fry the vegetables for 2 minutes. Do not forget to stir the vegetables constantly. Next, you should move the contents of the frying pan into the crock pot. At the same time, place mussels, scallops, and shrimps in the crock pot. After that, you should add the fish broth, parsley, and tomatoes. Now, close the lid of the pan tightly and cook the stew on low power for 4.5-5 hours or on strong power for 2-2.5 hours. Well done! Serve immediately!

Enjoy your meal!

12.Squids with sour cream and garlic

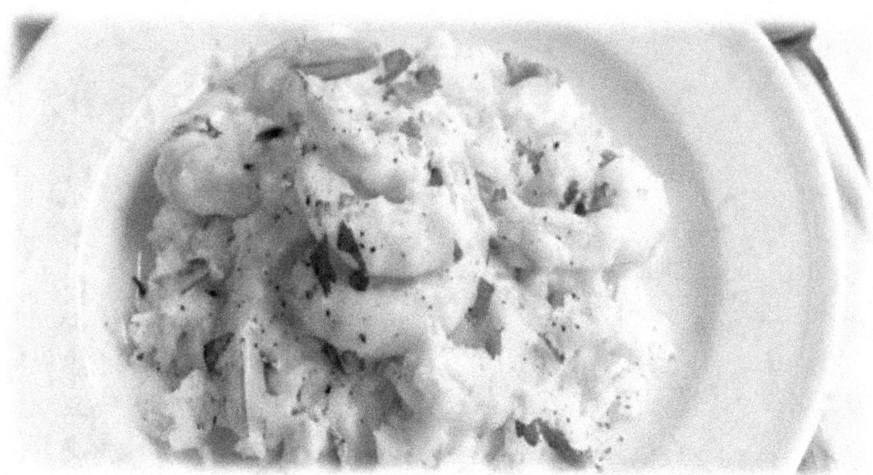

Ingredients (6 servings):

- 250 g of fresh squids
- 50 g of sour cream
- 1 clove of garlic
- fresh dill to taste
- salt to taste
- pepper black ground to taste

Cooking instruction:

As a first step, you need to wash the squids and put them in boiling water. Then you can remove the skin of the squids. Additionally, squids can be boiled in salted water for 5 minutes and then can move them to a colander. Now you can slice the squids into small pieces. At the same time, you should peel the garlic, wash it and finely chop. Do not forget to chop the fresh dill finely. After that, you should put the sliced squids, garlic and dill in a crock pot and fill it with sour cream. Next, add salt and pepper to taste. Mix the ingredients thoroughly and close the lid tightly. You should cook on low power for 4.5-5 hours or on strong power for 2-2.5 hours. Well done! Serve immediately!

Enjoy your meal!

13.Shrimp with lemon and herbs

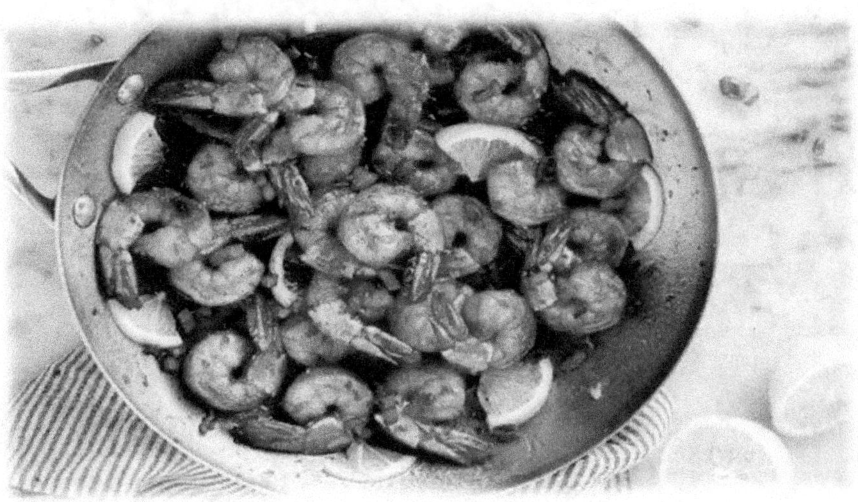

Ingredients (7 servings):

- 1 kg of shrimp
- 6 tablespoons of olive oil
- 3 cloves of pressed garlic
- 50 ml of lemon juice
- sliced lemon
- black pepper to taste
- any fresh herbs to taste

Cooking instruction:

 As a first step, you should place olive oil, lime juice, pressed garlic, and sliced lemon in a bowl to make a marinade for shrimp. Then stir them thoroughly. After that, place shrimp in the bowl with a marinade. Then, put the bowl in the refrigerator for 30 minutes. In 30 minutes, remove the bowl from refrigerator and leave it at room temperature for 15 minutes. After that, you should place the shrimp in the crock pot. You should cook the shrimp for about 2-2.5 hours. Well done! In addition, use fresh herbs to your taste.

Enjoy your meal!

14.Tuna broth with spices

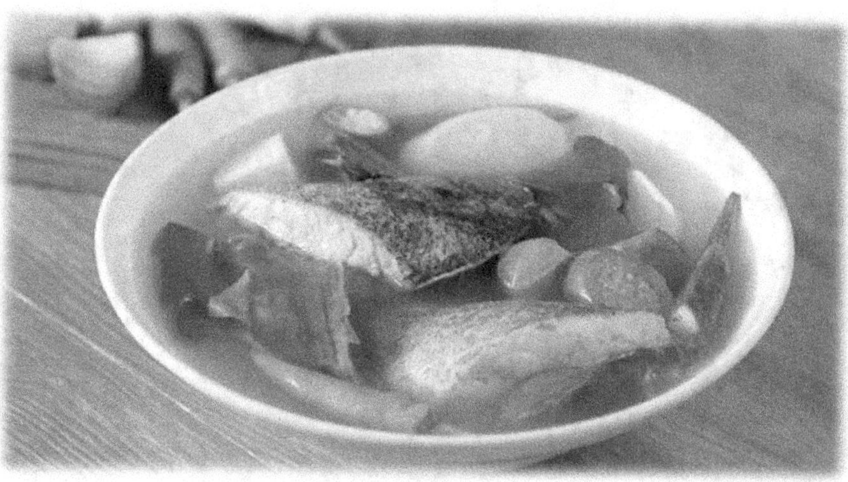

Ingredients (12 servings):

- 400 g of tuna
- 1 onion
- 1 lemon
- 1 tomato
- 4 tablespoons of olive oil
- 10 g of bay leaves
- 1 hot pepper
- 1 clove of garlic
- thyme to taste
- dill to taste
- coriander to taste
- ginger ground to taste
- salt to taste

Cooking instruction:

As a first step, you should divide the fish into large pieces. Then you should place the onions, tomatoes, spices, chopped herbs, hot pepper and water in the crock pot. Stir all ingredients thoroughly. You should cook the fish for about 2-2.5 hours. After that, remove the boiled fish and herbs from the crock pot. The fish should cool down, and then remove the bones from the meat. Then place the fish meat and crushed garlic in the broth. After that, you can add lemon juice. Well done!

Bon Appetite!

15.Scallops with lemon and spices

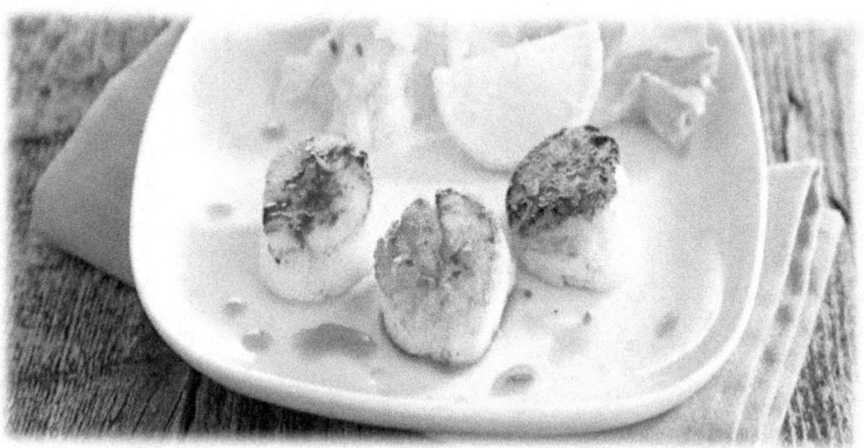

Ingredients (7 servings):

- 200 g of scallops
- 150 ml of water or clear vegetable soup
- 50 g of lemon juice
- oregano to taste
- freshly ground pepper to taste
- salt to taste
- sesame seeds to taste

Cooking instruction:

In the first instance, you should wash and dry the scallops. Then you can add salt, pepper, and oregano. You need to distribute the spices evenly over the surface. Then, pour water or clear vegetable soup in the crock pot and place the scallops there. After that, you should close the crock pot with a lid tightly and cook the scallops on low power for 4.5-5 hours or on strong power for 2-2.5 hours. Well done! Now, you can add the butter and lemon juice. Serve immediately!

Enjoy your meal!

16.Boiled lobsters with herbs

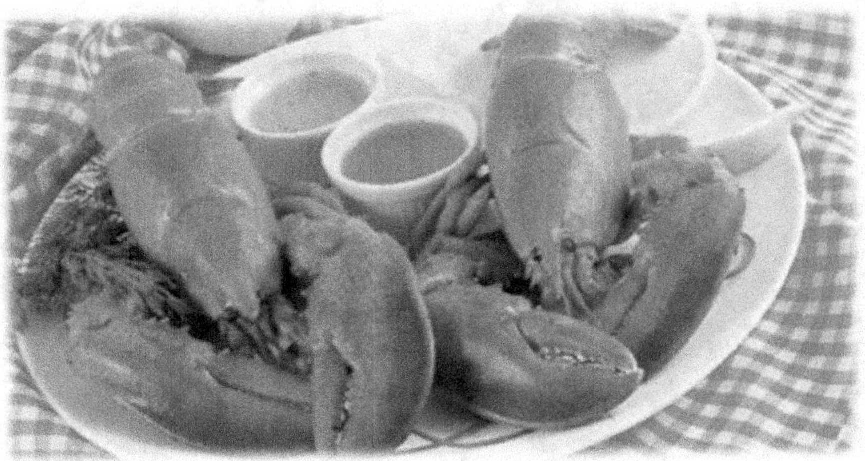

Ingredients (8 servings):

- 6-7 lobsters
- 1-2 cloves garlic
- 2 tablespoons of olive oil
- 1 tablespoon of soy sauce
- 250 ml of water or clear vegetable soup
- salt to taste
- black pepper to taste
- a few twigs of coriander
- a few twigs of parsley
- 1 tablespoon of lemon juice

Cooking instruction

As a first step, you should chop the fresh coriander and parsley. After that put chopped cilantro, parsley, crushed garlic, olive oil, soy sauce, lemon juice, salt and pepper in a deep bowl. Then stir the sauce thoroughly. It must be homogeneous. Now, you should place the lobsters on a flat dish. Now, you can place them in the deep bowl filled with marinade. After that, leave the lobsters to marinate for about 20 minutes. Well done! At the same time, you should fill the crock pot with water or clear vegetable soup. Place the lobsters in the pot and close them with a lid tightly. You should cook the lobsters on low power for 4.5-5 hours or on strong power for 2-2.5 hours. Serve immediately!

Enjoy your meal!

17.Korean mussels with spices

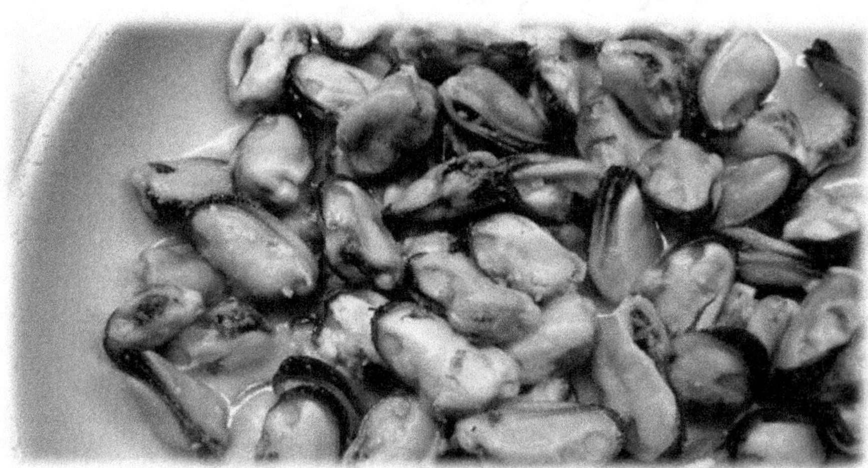

Ingredients (10 servings):

- 500 g of frozen mussels
- 3 onions
- 6 tablespoons of soy sauce
- 1 lemon
- ground nutmeg to taste
- salt to taste
- ground black pepper to taste
- ground red pepper to taste
- coriander powder to taste

Cooking instruction

In the first instance, you should defrost and wash the mussels well. Then place them in a crock pot. Close the mussels with a lid tightly. You should cook the mussels on low power for 4.5-5 hours or on strong power for 2-2.5 hours. At the same time, you should cut the onion and place it in a bowl. Then add lemon juice and mix well. Leave the bow to marinate for 10 minutes. Now you should make a mussel sauce. Then, pour soy sauce into a deep frying pan. Next, you should add lemon juice, red and black pepper, nutmeg and coriander. Stir all ingredients and put the frying pan on a medium heat. The sauce should be hot. However, you should not boil the sauce. At the same time, add boiled mussels to the sliced onion. After that, pour over sauce and mix well. After that, put the boiled mussels in the fridge for a few hours. Well done!
    Enjoy your meal!

18.Thai curry soup with seafood

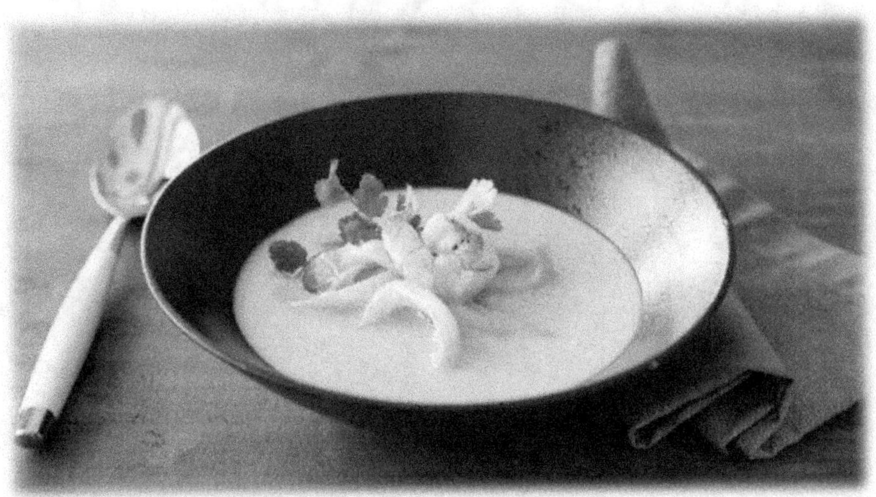

Ingredients (10 servings):

- 150 ml of clear vegetable soup
- 150 ml low fat cream
- 1 tablespoon of yellow curry paste
- 15 g of lemongrass herbs
- 3-4 shrimps size
- 3-4 rings of calamari
- salt to taste
- black pepper to taste
- 1-2 sprigs of coriander

Cooking instruction

As a first step, you should put the seafood in the crock pot. Then add the clear vegetable soup, curry paste, and lemongrass. Mix thoroughly all ingredients with a whisk until dissolved. After that, you should add salt and pepper to your taste. Stir the mass again. Close the seafood with a lid tightly. Well done! You should cook the seafood on low power for 4.5-5 hours or on strong power for 2-2.5 hours. Finally, you can decorate the dish with sprigs of coriander.

Enjoy your meal!

19.Stewed salmon with spices

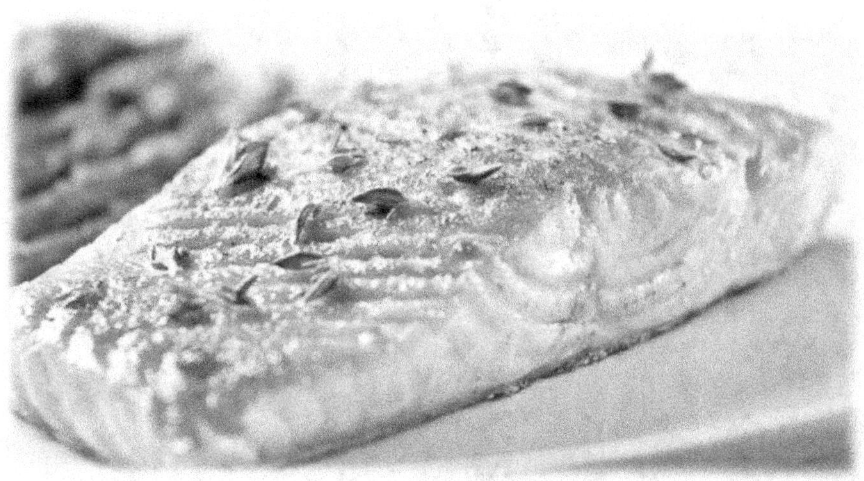

Ingredients (11 servings):

- salmon fillet
- 150 ml of sesame oil
- 150 ml of soy sauce
- 1 teaspoon of crushed garlic
- ½ teaspoon of ground dried ginger
- ½ teaspoon of dried basil
- 1 ½ teaspoon of dried oregano
- ¼ teaspoon of dried thyme
- ½ teaspoon of dried rosemary
- ½ teaspoon of dried tarragon
- 70 g of green onions

Cooking instruction

In the first instance, you should cook the marinade. Place crushed garlic, ginger, basil, oregano, thyme, rosemary, tarragon, soy sauce and sesame oil in a deep bowl. You should stir all spices thoroughly. After that, take the deep bowl filled with marinade and put the fish in it. Now, you should leave the deep bowl in the fridge for 1 hour or even more. Well done! Finally, you can place the fish in the crock pot. Do not forget to pour the marinade in the crock pot. Then you should close the pot with a lid tightly. You should cook the salmon on low power for 4.5-5 hours or on strong power for 2-2.5 hours. In the end, you can decorate the salmon with fresh herbs to your taste.

Enjoy your meal!

Soups & Cream Soups

20.Vegetarian cream soup

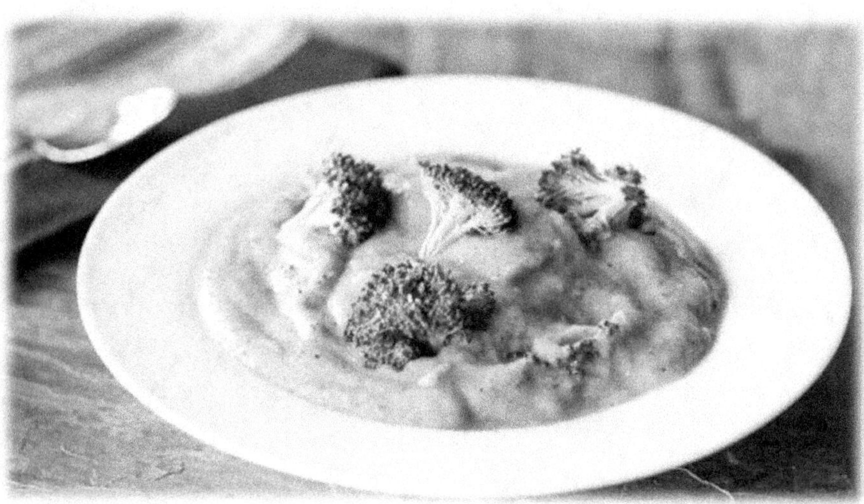

Ingredients (5 servings):

- 1kg of broccoli
- 6 glasses of clear vegetable broth
- 1/2 of onion
- 1 tablespoon of olive oil
- 1/2 teaspoon of salt
- olive oil

Cooking instruction:

As a first step, you should cut broccoli into pieces. Then you should finely chop the onion. After that, heat the olive oil in a frying pan and fry chopped onion for 10 minutes on a low heat. At the same time, you can pour vegetable broth in a crock pot. Then, you can place there all fried vegetables, and add salt to taste. Stir well. Then you should close the pot with a lid tightly. You should cook the vegetables on low power for 4.5-5 hours or on strong power for 2-2.5 hours. After that, pour the contents of the crock pot into a blender and grind all the ingredients until a homogeneous mass is obtained. Well done! You can decorate the soup with fresh herbs or boiled broccoli at will. Serve immediately!

Enjoy your meal!

21.Pumpkin cream soup

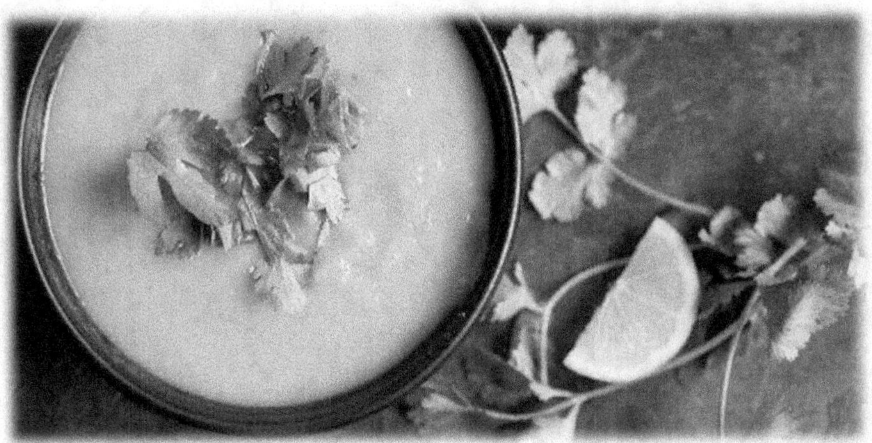

Ingredients (8 servings):

- 500 g of pumpkin flesh
- 1 onion
- 1 garlic
- 1 l of chicken broth
- salt to taste
- black pepper to taste
- any herbs to taste
- lemon juice to taste

Cooking instruction

In the first instance, you should wash the vegetables. After that, cut pumpkin flesh and onions into pieces and put them in a crock pot. In addition, add the chicken broth to the pot. Then you should close the pot with a lid tightly. You should cook the vegetables on low power for 4.5-5 hours or on strong power for 2-2.5 hours. All the ingredients should become soft. Then you should add the chopped fresh herbs to your taste and garlic to the vegetable broth. Stir the broth well. Now, you can pour the content of the crock pot in a blender. Next, you should grind all the boiled ingredients in the blender. Well done! Do not forget to decorate the cream soup with fresh herbs. Serve immediately.

Enjoy your meal!

22.Vegetable cream- soup

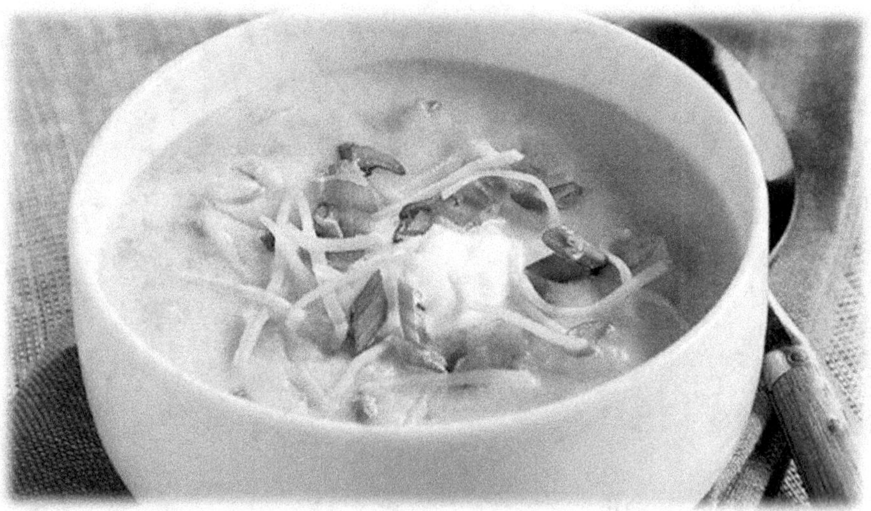

Ingredients (13 servings):

- sliced bacon
- 2 tablespoons of butter
- 2 cloves of garlic
- 1 onion
- 1 celery
- 4 cups of chicken broth
- 1 cup of milk
- grated cheese to your taste
- cauliflower
- a bay leaf
- black pepper to taste
- fresh herbs to taste

Cooking instruction:

In the first instance, you should place sliced bacon in the pan and fry them for 10 minutes until they become golden. After that, place fried slices of bacon on a paper towel. Then, you should slice onion, celery, cauliflower, and garlic. Next, add the chopped vegetables to the melted butter in a pan. Stir the sliced vegetables well. After that, you should add cauliflower and a bay leaf. At the same time, pour the chicken broth and milk in the crock pot. Finally, you can add fried vegetables in the crock pot. Stir the ingredients thoroughly. Then you should close the pot with a lid tightly. You should cook the vegetables on low power for 4.5-5 hours or on strong power for 2-2.5 hours. Well done! Now, you can add pepper to taste. Do not forget to decorate your cream-soup with fresh herbs, grated cheese and fried slices of bacon. Serve immediately!

Enjoy your meal!

23.Chicken soup with cream cheese

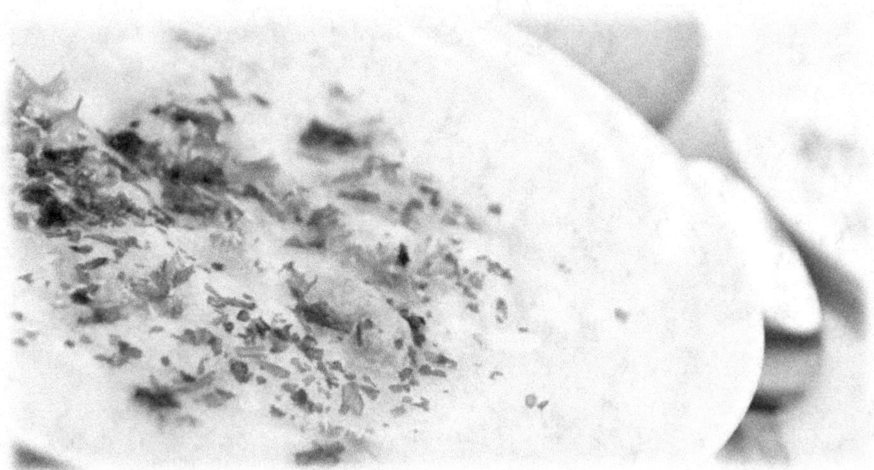

Ingredients (14 servings):

- 300 g of chicken fillet
- 50 g of bell pepper
- 30 g of chopped onion
- 100 g of cream cheese
- 25 g butter
- black pepper to taste
- 2 g of bay leaves
- salt to taste
- 1.5 liters of water
- any chopped fresh herbs

Cooking instruction

As a first step, you should place the chicken in the crock pot. Then you should add the bay leaf, and black pepper to taste. Then you should close the pot with a lid tightly. You should cook the chicken on low power for 4.5-5 hours or on strong power for 2-2.5 hours.

At the same time, chop the bell pepper and onions finely. After that, place the chopped bell pepper, and onions in a frying pan with melted butter. You should fry vegetables for 10 minutes. After that, place the fried vegetables in the crock pot and cook at least for 2-2.5 hours. Well done! Now you can add cream cheese to the chicken soup. The cheese should completely melt. After that, decorate the chicken soup with fresh herbs. Serve immediately!

Enjoy your meal!

24. Beef soup with fresh herbs

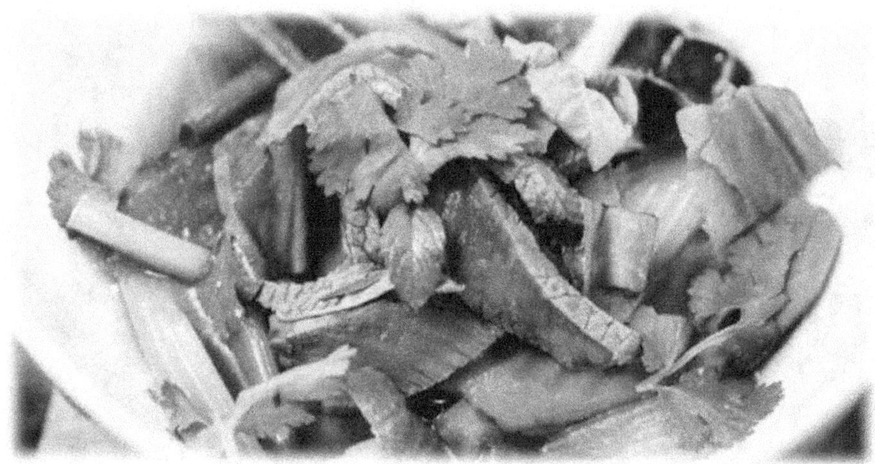

Ingredients (7 servings):

- 1 kg of beef
- leeks
- 1 fresh onion
- 3 g of bay leaves
- black pepper to taste
- salt to taste
- any chopped fresh herbs

Cooking instruction:

In the first instant, you should put the sliced beef in the crock pot. Then pour three liters of water. After that, wash leeks thoroughly and cut them into large pieces. Also, chop the onion. Now, you can place all cut vegetables and bay leaves in the pot. In addition, add salt and black pepper to taste. Stir all ingredients well. Now, you should cover the crock pot with a lid tightly and cook the beef soup on low power for 4.5-5 hours or on strong power for 2-2.5 hours. Well done! Serve immediately!

Enjoy your meal!

25.Georgian vegetable soup

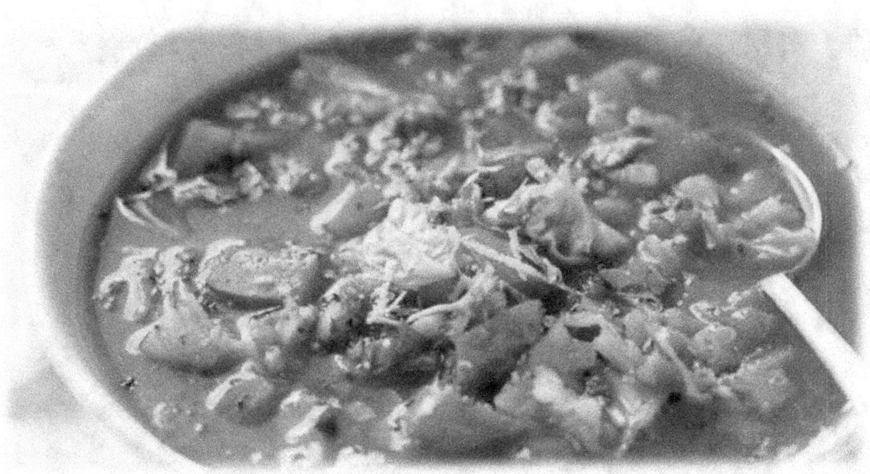

Ingredients (12 servings):

- 1 eggplant
- 100 g of pumpkin
- sliced cabbage
- 10 cherry tomatoes
- 1 onion
- 1 clove of garlic
- 2 bay leaves
- 2-3 tablespoons of olive oil
- a few sprigs of green basil
- salt to taste
- black pepper to taste

Cooking instruction:

As a first step, you should cut eggplant, cabbage, and pumpkin into small slices. Then place all the sliced vegetables in the crock pot. Then cover the pot with a lid and cook the vegetable broth on low power for 4.5-5 hours or on strong power for 2-2.5 hours. After that, you should chop the onions and garlic finely. Next, heat olive oil in a frying pan and fry onion and garlic for 5-7 minutes. Stir thoroughly. After that cut the cherry tomatoes into halves and simmer them for 3 minutes in the same frying pan. Now, you can add salt, pepper to taste and cook the vegetables for 12-15 minutes. Finally, you should combine fried vegetables with vegetable broth. Stir thoroughly. Well done! Serve immediately!

Enjoy your meal!

26.Curry cream soup with salmon

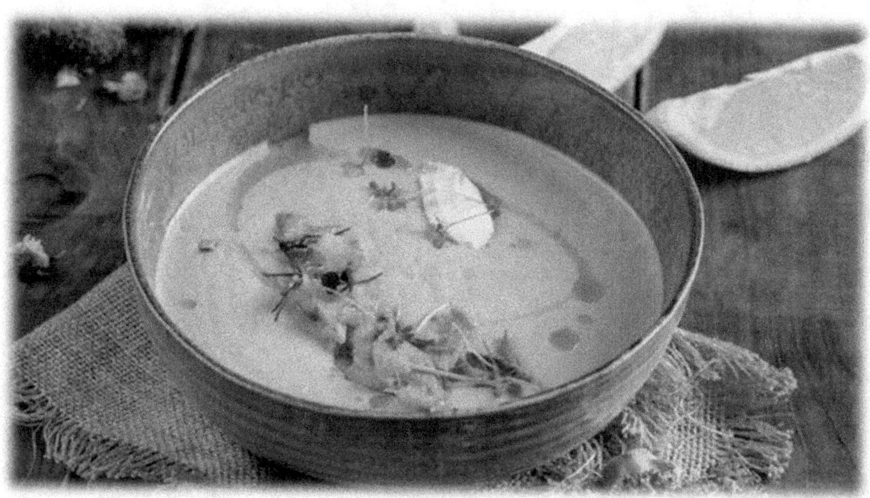

Ingredients (11 servings):

- 400 g of broccoli
- grated cheese
- 150 g of salmon
- 200 ml of cream
- 1 teaspoon of butter
- 1 onions
- curry to taste
- salt to taste
- black pepper to taste
- 1l of chicken broth
- any chopped fresh herbs

Cooking instruction

In the first instant, you should melt the butter on the bottom of the pan and put rings of onions. You should fry rings of onions until they get golden. Then pour the chicken broth in the crock pot. After, add the fried rings of onions, chopped broccoli, and curry. Then cover the pot with a lid and cook the vegetable broth on low power for 4.5-5 hours or on strong power for 2-2.5 hours. Well done! Then, you should let the soup cool down for 20 minutes. Next, you can use the blender to grind all the ingredients. After grinding, put crushed ingredients in the pan on a medium heat. Next, you should add the cream and cheese. Stir the soup thoroughly. After boiling, you should use the blender to mix everything again. After all, you will get the creamy consistency. The curry soup should be served immediately. Do not forget to decorate the dish with sliced salmon and fresh herbs to your taste.

Enjoy your meal!

27.Spinach cream soup

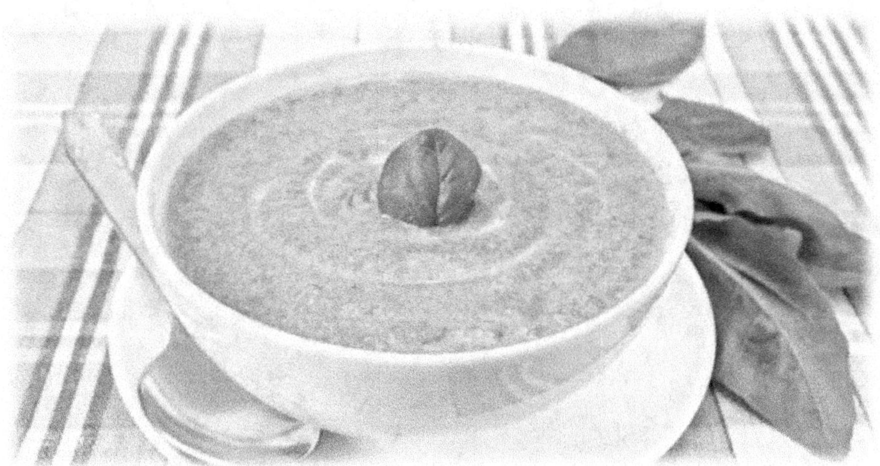

Ingredients (7 servings):

- 1 l of chicken broth
- sliced onion
- 500 g spinach
- 100 g cream
- 1 tablespoon of butter
- black ground pepper to taste
- salt to taste

Cooking instruction

As a first step, you should place the chopped onions in a pan with melted butter. You should cook for 15 minutes. Then place fried onions in the crock pot and pour the chicken broth. After that, you can add the finely chopped spinach, salt, and pepper to your taste. Then cover the pot with a lid and cook the vegetable broth on low power for 4.5-5 hours or on strong power for 2-2.5 hours. Well done! In the end, you should pour the broth in a blender. Then grind all the ingredients thoroughly. Then return the broth to the crock pot and add the cream. You should cook the soup at least for one hour. Well done! Do not forget to decorate the dish with a sprig of spinach. Serve immediately!

Enjoy your meal!

Meat dishes

28.Chicken cutlets with herbs

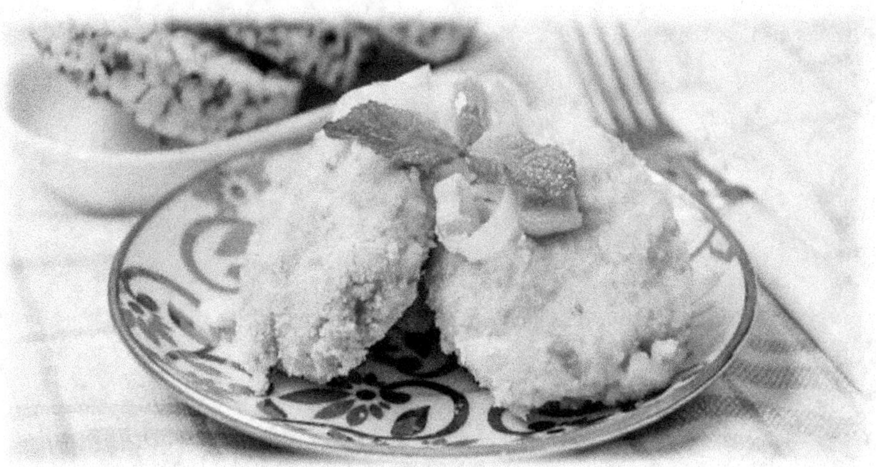

Ingredients (6 servings):

- 800 g of chicken mince
- 1/3 cup of milk
- 1 onion
- salt to taste
- black ground pepper to taste
- any fresh herbs to taste

Cooking instruction:

As a first step, you should grind an onion in the blender. After that, you should add the onions to the mince, and mix thoroughly. Then add the finely chopped herbs, salt, and pepper to taste. Stir well again. After that, you should form cutlets. Well done! Now, you can place all cutlets in the crock pot. Then cover the crock pot with a lid and cook the chicken cutlets on low power for 4.5-5 hours or on strong power for 2-2.5 hours. Serve immediately!
   Enjoy your meal!

29. Turkey breast with vegetables

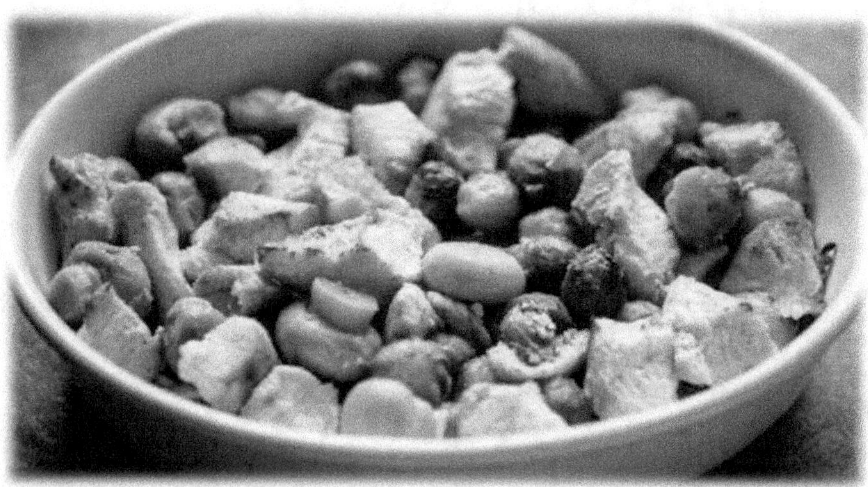

Ingredients (10 servings):

- 500 g of turkey breast
- 100 g of mushrooms
- 200 g of Brussels sprout
- 1 onion
- 1 teaspoon of walnuts
- spices to taste
- vegetable oil
- fresh herbs to taste
- salt to taste
- black pepper to taste

Cooking instruction

As a first step, you should chop the turkey breast into small pieces and place them in a deep bowl. Then chop an onion into rings and add to the turkey meat. After that, add salt and black pepper to taste. Stir thoroughly and place a bowl of meat in the refrigerator at least for one hour. After that, you should put the content of the bowl in the crock pot. In addition, put their mushrooms, one teaspoon of ground walnuts, Brussels sprout, spices and fresh herbs to taste. Then add 100 ml of water and stir well. Then cover the crock pot with a lid and cook on low power for 4.5-5 hours or on strong power for 2-2.5 hours. At the end of cooking, do not forget to decorate the dish with fresh herbs. Well done! Serve immediately.

Enjoy your meal!

30.Chicken stewed with vegetables

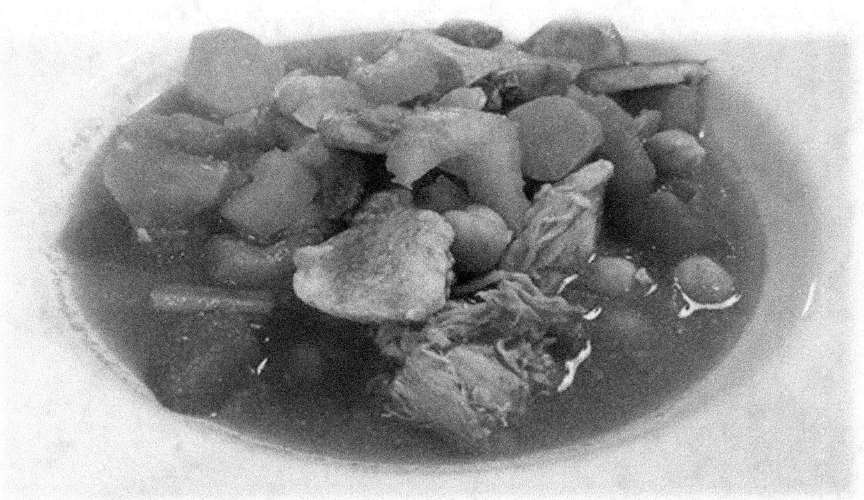

Ingredients (9 servings):

- 1 kg of chicken fillet
- 500 ml of water
- 2 tomatoes
- 2 bell peppers
- 1 onion
- 2 cloves of garlic
- any fresh herbs to taste
- salt to taste
- paprika to taste

Cooking instruction:

In the first instance, you should cut the chicken fillet into cubes. After that, remove all seeds from bell peppers and chop them finely. Now you can chop tomatoes, onion, and garlic. Then pour 500 ml of water in the crock pot and place where all the ingredients except parsley. Then add salt and paprika to taste. Stir all ingredients thoroughly. Then cover the crock pot with a lid and cook chicken with vegetables on low power for 4.5-5 hours or on strong power for 2-2.5 hours. Well done! Now you can decorate the dish with fresh parsley. Serve immediately!

Enjoy your meal!

31.Pork stewed with lemon and sesame

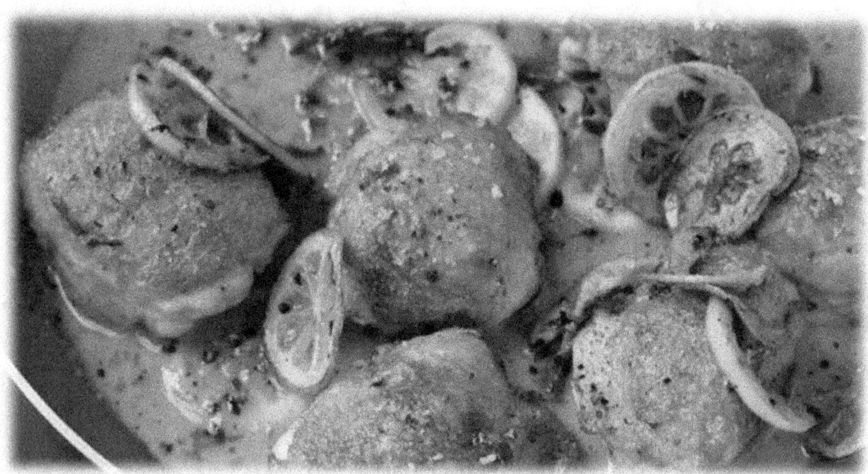

Ingredients (9 servings):

- 450 g of pork
- 200 g of onions
- 2 tablespoons of sesame seeds
- 100 g of coriander
- salt to taste
- black pepper to taste
- 2 tablespoons of lemon juice
- sliced lemon
- olive oil

Cooking instruction

As a first step, you should cut pork into small pieces. Then cook the marinade by mixing olive oil, juice and lemon peel. Add the marinade to the pork and mix thoroughly. After that, you should cover the pork with a lid and put it in the refrigerator for 30 minutes. At the same time, you should fry lightly sesame seeds in a dry frying pan. Then pour the olive oil and add finely chopped onions. Fry the onion until it is soft. Then place the pork in the crock pot. In addition, you should place all content of the frying pan and sliced lemon in the crock pot. Then cover the crock pot with a lid and cook the pork on low power for 4.5-5 hours or on strong power for 2-2.5 hours. Well done! In addition, you can decorate the pork with fresh herbs. Serve immediately!

Enjoy your meal!

32. Pork meatballs

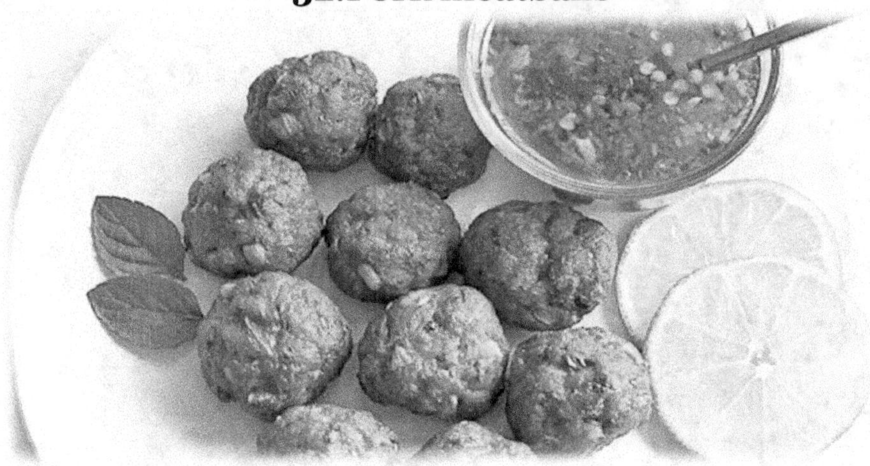

Ingredients (7 servings):

- 1 kg of ground pork
- 200 g of breadcrumbs
- 2 eggs
- 5 tablespoons of olive oil
- fresh herbs to taste
- pepper to taste
- other spices to taste

Cooking instruction:

In the first instance, you should mix ground pork, breadcrumbs, eggs and 5 tablespoons of olive oil in a large bowl. Then you should mix the ingredients thoroughly. After that, you can add the pepper and other species to your taste and stir all ingredients well. If you want, you can add the chopped fresh herbs to the ground pork. Now, you can form meatballs. After, you should place them in the crock pot and add a little water. After that, you should close the crock pot and cook meatballs on low power or 5-6 hours at a strong power 2.5-3 hours. Well done! Serve immediately.

    Enjoy your meal!

33. Boiled dinner with pork

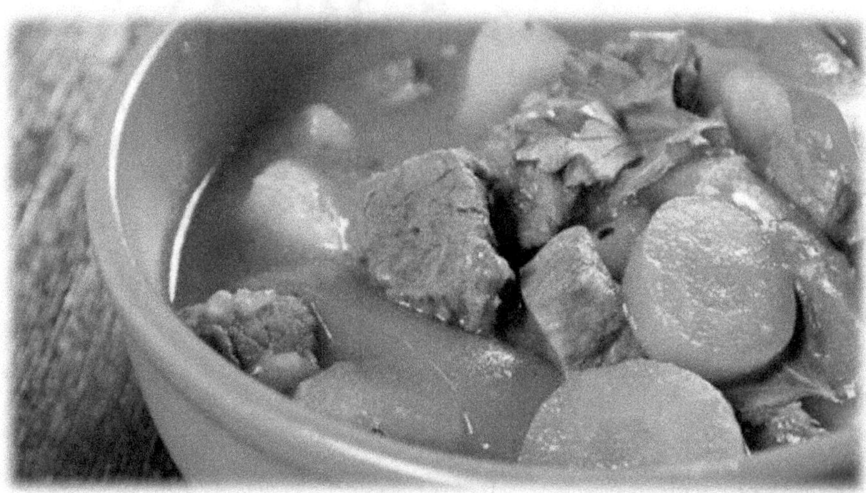

Ingredients (11 servings):

- 500 g of pork
- 2 tomatoes
- 2 bell peppers
- curry spices to taste
- black pepper to taste
- 2 garlics
- 1 onion
- fresh herbs to taste
- salt to taste
- 250 ml of water or vegetable broth

Cooking instruction

As a first step, you should chop the pork into medium pieces. After that, you should add salt and black pepper to taste. Stir well. After that, you should chop the onions, tomatoes and bell peppers into small cubes and add them to the pork. Stir the ingredients thoroughly. Then add curry spice, water or vegetable broth and add salt to taste. Then cover the crock pot with a lid and cook the pork on low power for 4.5-5 hours or on strong power for 2-2.5 hours. Well done! Serve immediately!

Enjoy your meal!

34.Duck stewed with vegetables

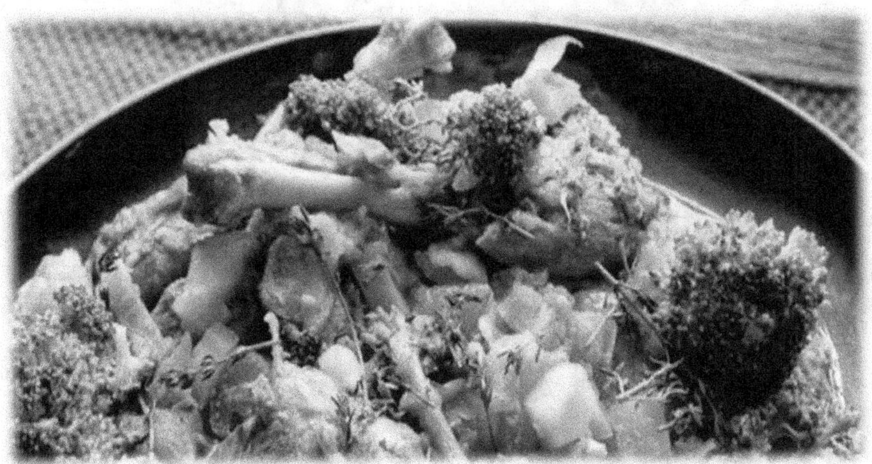

Ingredients (11 servings):

- about 1 kg of duck leg
- 1 onion
- 150 g of broccoli
- 200 g of sour cabbage
- 1 teaspoon of dried herbs
- ½ teaspoon of black pepper
- 1 teaspoon of bayberry
- 2 g of bay leaves
- salt to taste

Cooking instruction

In the first instance, you should cut off excess fat from duck legs. Next, cut duck fat and meat into pieces. After that, put duck fat and meat in the crock pot. Then cut the onions and broccoli into half rings. Add the chopped vegetables to the duck meat. After that, please add salt and pepper to taste. Next, you should sour cabbage in the frying pan. In addition, you should add black ground pepper, bayberry, and bay leaf, spicy dried herbs, for example, dill, parsley, basil, and celery. Thoroughly mix all the ingredients. Then cover the crock pot with a lid and cook the pork on low power for 4.5-5 hours or on strong power for 2-2.5 hours. Well done! Serve immediately!

Enjoy your meal!

35. Duck stewed with orange

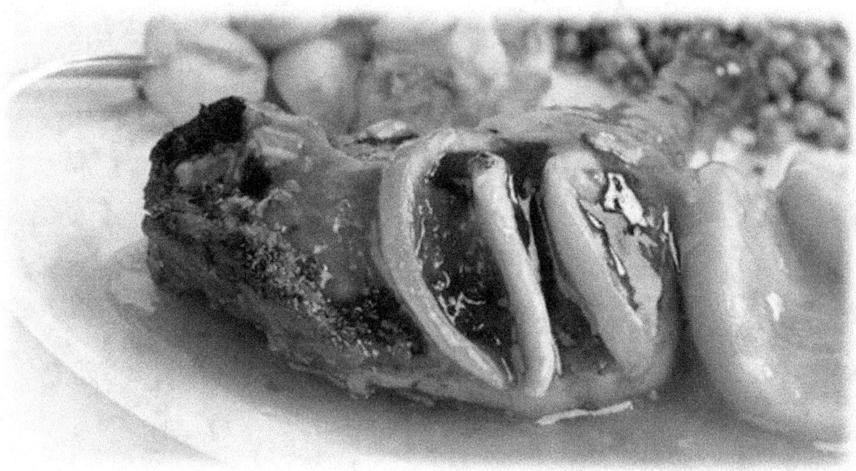

Ingredients (9 servings):

- about 1 kg of duck leg
- 150 g of boiled white mushrooms
- 2 oranges
- 1 onions
- 200 ml of cream
- spices to taste
- salt to taste
- any fresh herbs to taste

Cooking instruction

As a first step, you should cut off excess fat from duck legs. Next, cut duck fat and meat into pieces. After that, put duck fat and meat in a deep bowl. Then, chop oranges, boiled white mushrooms, and onions into half rings and add to the chopped meat. Add the spices and salt to your taste. Stir thoroughly and place the bowl in the refrigerator for 1 hour. After that, replace the content of the bowl in the crock pot. Then cover the crock pot with a lid and cook the pork on low power for 4.5-5 hours or on strong power for 2-2.5 hours. Well done! Serve immediately!

Enjoy your meal!

36.Stuffed eggplants with herbs

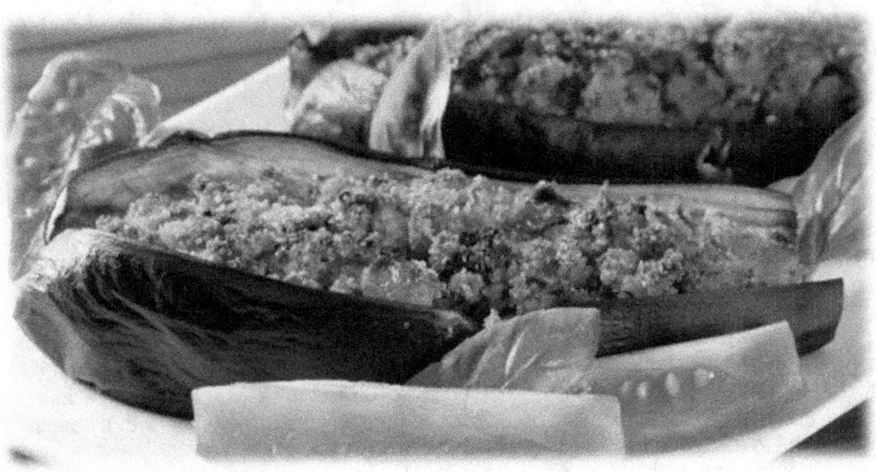

Ingredients (9 servings):

- 4 eggplants
- 500 g of minced beef
- 250 g of tomato sauce
- 1 onion
- chopped fresh herbs to your taste
- 2 cloves garlic
- salt to taste
- 1 cup of water or clear vegetable soup
- pepper to taste

Cooking instruction:

As a first step, you should remove eggplants flesh. Now, you can peel onion and garlic and finely chop them. In addition, chop any fresh herbs to your taste. Stir the minced meat, pepper, onion, garlic, and tomato sauce. By the way, instead of beef meat, you can use any minced meat. Then you should add salt, pepper to taste and stir well. Next, fill the eggplants with minced beef. Finally, you can place the stuffed eggplants in the crock pot and add water or clear vegetable soup. After that, cover the crock pot with a lid and cook the eggplants for 6-7 hours. Well done! Serve immediately.

Enjoy your meal!

Conclusion

Eating habits play a major role in the development of overweight and obesity. Most eating habits are passed from generation to generation. Children, who eat fast food and drink soda, will pass on these traditions to their future families. Being overweight can have a significant impact on health. The overweight problems frequently lead to serious health consequences such as cardiovascular diseases, mainly heart disease and stroke, and diabetes, muscular-skeletal injuries, such as osteoarthritis, and some cancers, for instance, cancer of the endometrium, breast death, and colorectal carcinoma. These conditions cause premature death or disability. Not everyone knows that the risk of health problems starts when someone is only slightly overweight and the risk increases with increasing weight. Many of the conditions I have listed cause long-term suffering to people and their families.

For the very reason, many modern people are concerned about how quickly to lose weight without harm to health. Moreover, is it possible? The answer to this question is very simple. The diet without harm to health should be based on the principles of healthy eating. In addition to it, you need to take the first step towards your health and happiness of your family. I am sure that my book will be useful for you. Doubtless, you will find for yourself many useful and tasty healthy dishes on the pages of this book. I wish you with pleasure to pass the way to ideal health, optimal weight, and inexhaustible vital energy.

In conclusion, I would like to add that we are the creators of our own destiny. Moreover, our life, our health depends only on us. Remember that early diagnosis and detection of the cause of overweight greatly facilitate the treatment of complications or prevent their occurrence. Take care of yourself and love your body.

Good luck!

Author's Afterthoughts

Thanks ever so much to each of my cherished readers for investing the time read this book!

I know you could have picked from many other books but you chose this one. So a big thanks for downloading this book and reading all way to the end.

If you enjoyed this book or received value from it, I'd like to ask you for a favor. Please take a few minutes to post an honest and heartfelt review on Amazon.com Your support does make a difference and to benefit other people.

Text Copyright © Joshua Chase

Legal & Disclaimer

The information contained in this book and its contents is not designed to replace or take the place of any form of medical or professional advice; and is not meant to replace the need for independent medical, financial, legal or other professional advice or services, as may be required. The content and information in this book has been provided for educational and entertainment purposes only.

The content and information contained in this book has been compiled from sources deemed reliable, and it is accurate to the best of the Author's knowledge, information and belief. However, the Author cannot guarantee its accuracy and validity and cannot be held liable for any errors and/or omissions. Further, changes are periodically made to this book as and when needed. Where appropriate and/or necessary, you must consult a professional (including but not limited to your doctor, attorney, financial advisor or such other professional advisor) before using any of the suggested remedies, techniques, or information in this book.

Upon using the contents and information contained in this book, you agree to hold harmless the Author from and against any damages, costs, and expenses, including any legal fees potentially resulting from the application of any of the information provided by this book. This disclaimer applies to any loss, damages or injury caused by the use and application, whether directly or indirectly, of any advice or information presented, whether for breach of contract, tort, negligence, personal injury, criminal intent, or under any other cause of action.

You agree to accept all risks of using the information presented inside this book.

You agree that by continuing to read this book, where appropriate and/or necessary, you shall consult a professional (including but not limited to your doctor, attorney, or financial advisor or such other advisor as needed) before using any of the suggested remedies, techniques, or information in this book.